A Recipe Book for Tutors

Teaching the Kinesthetic Learner

Cynthia Parsons

Rowman & Littlefield Education
Lanham, Maryland • Toronto • Plymouth, UK
2008

Published in the United States of America
by Rowman & Littlefield Education
A Division of Rowman & Littlefield Publishers, Inc.
A wholly owned subsidiary of The Rowman & Littlefield Publishing Group, Inc.
4501 Forbes Boulevard, Suite 200, Lanham, Maryland 20706
www.rowmaneducation.com

Estover Road
Plymouth PL6 7PY
United Kingdom

Copyright © 2008 by Cynthia Parsons

All rights reserved. No part of this publication may be reproduced,
stored in a retrieval system, or transmitted in any form or by any
means, electronic, mechanical, photocopying, recording, or otherwise,
without the prior permission of the publisher.

British Library Cataloguing in Publication Information Available

Library of Congress Cataloging-in-Publication Data

Parsons, Cynthia.
  A recipe book for tutors : teaching the kinesthetic learner / Cynthia Parsons.
    p. cm.
  ISBN-13: 978-1-57886-790-5 (hardcover : alk. paper)
  ISBN-13: 978-1-57886-791-2 (pbk. : alk. paper)
  ISBN-10: 1-57886-790-8 (hardcover : alk. paper)
  ISBN-10: 1-57886-791-6 (pbk. : alk. paper)
   1. Activity programs in education. 2. Teaching. 3. Kinesiology. 4. Mind and body. 5. Learning, Psychology of. I. Title.
  LB1027.25.P37   2008
  371.39'4—dc22   2007046650

∞ ™ The paper used in this publication meets the minimum requirements of
American National Standard for Information Sciences—Permanence of Paper for
Printed Library Materials, ANSI/NISO Z39.48-1992. Manufactured in the United
States of America.

Contents

Foreword	*Mark B. Perkins*	v
Preface		vii
Step 1	Begin the New Learning Arrangement	1
Step 2	Jump into Lesson 2	7
Step 3	Tackle Lesson 3	17
Step 4	Take Stock	25
Step 5	Dictate a Story	39
Step 6	Season with Mathematics throughout the Lessons	49
Step 7	Garnish with the Arts throughout the Lessons	101
Step 8	Stop Reading Aloud	111
Step 9	Support Your Pupil's Success	119

Foreword

As an educator for the past 38 years and head of The Forman School, a college preparatory school for students with learning differences, I applaud Cynthia Parsons's vision of providing a book to teach the unsuccessful reader. Time and again, we at Forman find students who can succeed if they are taught with the proper methods. Every student's brain is different, and not all students are "wired" to pick up reading naturally. This doesn't mean they are unintelligent; it just means they learn differently. Cynthia Parsons has pulled together the many kinesthetic teaching methods into a comprehensive plan to guarantee your student's success.

Cynthia Parsons knows the truth about teaching: most successful students teach themselves the skills acquired in school. This is not to say that the teacher isn't important, but that most skills are self-evident to the successful learner. Teachers introduce the information and provide exercises for repetition, and the student learns. Once the successful learner receives the explanation, he or she is off and running with the new skill. Such is reading.

This book is what every elementary teacher needs. It is a "how-to" book for teaching reading to the previously unsuccessful reader. Cynthia Parsons writes her book the way a good football coach writes a training manual. Skills are broken down into steps that every child of normal intelligence can understand and perform.

After presenting a comprehensive overview, she lays down some ground rules. Most important is determining your student's learning style: visual, auditory, kinesthetic. Then she makes it clear that it is the teacher's responsibility to teach the student—not the student's responsibility to figure out how to learn to read. Cynthia Parsons understands the unsuccessful learner and the psychological stumbling blocks that get in the way of the student's self-motivation. She says, "You . . . have to assure the pupil that the problem [is] not his/hers, but the fault of the teaching."

If all elementary teachers would adopt Cynthia Parsons's reading methodology, The Forman School might find itself without any students. At this point, however, we have a full and thriving school. We are proud of our students and alumni—one of whom is Cynthia Parsons.

Mark B. Perkins
Head of School
The Forman School
Litchfield, CT

Preface

The 8-, 9-, or 10-year-old of normal intelligence and vision who has not learned to read by the close of grade 3 needs special tutoring assistance. Think of how awful it would have been if you had been one of the few children who—all through primary school—didn't "catch on" to reading, even though teacher after teacher had tried to teach you. You might even have known by heart some of the storybooks that had been read to you, yet if you took the book and sat down by yourself with it, you couldn't tell by looking at them which word was which.

While there are several possible reasons why this experience is true for a few pupils, this book assumes that the struggling young reader doesn't learn primarily by sounding words or primarily by looking at words, but by feeling words, letters, and numbers; that is, he or she learns kinesthetically. This book also assumes that during the three critical years of basic schooling—in grades 1, 2, and 3—the nonreader was not given sufficient kinesthetic instruction.

Also, it is true that those who don't "catch on" to reading at what is considered to be the normal rate become both discouraged and humiliated and develop all sorts of avoidance behaviors just because they cannot keep up—as emerging readers—with their classmates.

The word "kinesthetic" has gone out of vogue in school settings. I recently bought a set of Uppercase Tactile Letters at a store full of teaching supplies. They are manuscript (not cursive), and the packet states that they are "sandpaper-textured letter cards." What I am calling "the kinesthetic way," some reading experts refer to as "tactile activities."

"Kinesthesia" is the noun; "kinesthetic," the adjective. Kinesthesia can be defined as sensation of movement from sensory nerve endings. The kinesthetic way of learning includes feeling while seeing and sounding. Learning to write the uppercase letter "A" by actually tracing with a finger of one's writing hand the sandpaper-textured letter "A" is a must for the kinesthetic learner.

If, instead of teaching reading to its pupils, a primary school spent comparable daily time for some 170 days a year teaching ice skating, and one or two of the members of the grade 1 class couldn't stay up on the skates after the first try, or the second try, or 170 tries, those non-skaters surely would have devised some very powerful avoidance strategies. But what is most significant is that the teachers might have "given up" on these pupils, lacking the understanding of how to teach them since they were not responding "normally."

Now picture an entire second year of minimum four hours a day for some 170 days, plus the teachers asking for daily "homework" time supervised by parents and guardians, and still no fluency of movement on those ice skates. Add the third year, and you get a glimpse of the forces attacking the nonreader.

If it was skating and you were the child who couldn't learn to skate, you'd probably destroy your skates (or hide them where they could not be found), or melt the ice!

And so it is for the nonreader. The child is frustrated; the teachers are puzzled if not humiliated; the parents are accused of not being supportive enough; and, as part of the downside of No Child Left Behind, the school administrators and teaching staff might be classified as "failing." In an extreme case, the school might have to close.

Clearly, finding the right method to teach each struggling pupil is essential. Of course, phonics will help—as will decoding, as will sight recognition—but two things are absolutely essential: (1) assuring the pupil that you can, in fact, teach him to read; and (2) that you will use the kinesthetic method as your primary teaching tool. You must shift the burden from the pupil to the tutor. The child must understand that it is your job to teach him or her to read and that you won't stop until you have succeeded.

To use the ice skating analogy once more: you would really have to be persuasive about your teaching skills to assure a non-skater that after three years of trying and failing, he or she could learn to skate.

You would have to assure the pupil that the problem was not his or hers, but the fault was with the teaching. You would have to admit that the method of instruction had been the wrong one and that now you can guarantee success by using correct teaching methods.

As every successful primary-level teacher knows, most of the pupils who become good readers quickly teach themselves to read. Just as the child with good balance glides off almost immediately after first putting on a pair of ice skates, so some first graders puzzle out the sound, look, and meaning of written words quickly and easily. We teachers like to think we should take some credit for pointing out sight-word commonalities and for providing phonics lessons, but in reality, we're just organizing practice time.

The child has figured it out through his or her individual learning style. Yes, we've helped in development of vocabulary and context—after all, the farm child needs help with city references and vice versa. But it is the child who actually does the "decoding" and "sounding" in order to become a fluent reader.

And now, let me make the following guarantee—the same guarantee that you should make with your "poor" reader: I promise you—you good and conscientious tutor—that you will learn from this book how to help the third and fourth graders still struggling with learning how to read, and you will be successful.

While you can teach them how to use their kinesthetic abilities to learn to read, it will, of course, take more than a year for them to "catch up" with their peers. But once they recognize that they are, in fact, reading, they will stop trying to "melt the ice" and devote themselves to catching up.

Through your excellent teaching, you will set them on the road to success. It is thrilling, exciting, and exacting work. But the reward is significant—not, of course, as much for you as for your pupil. You will have enormous satisfaction knowing that you have rescued someone who was in the final stages of both "giving up" and of being "given up."

This remedial teaching is next to impossible to do while instructing a classroom full of children. It requires a tutor (parent, college-level student teacher, guardian, retired teacher, caregiver) and a "recipe" book.

Why am I so sure you will succeed? I taught—with 100 percent success—in a private school and tutoring summer camp (Desert Sun in Idyllwild, California), mentored by a faculty made up of teachers trained in the kinesthetic method. As a novice in the UCLA clinic, I spent one summer tutoring a nonreader to read, supervised by Drs. Fernald and Sullivan and their staff of experts. I tutored fourth- and fifth-grade nonreaders within public school classrooms in North Adams and Westwood, Massachusetts, and Tarrytown, New York. And for 37 years I tutored individual children, "fixing" their individual stumbling blocks to learning.

My thesis for my master's degree in education was based on my experience tutoring a high school nonreader who went on to complete high school and earn a B.A. degree.

Before you take on a nonreader, let me ask you to take a few tests. You need to discover something about your own learning methods.

Test 1: Have a colleague or friend test your *sight recognition* and memory. Ask that 20 common objects be placed on a flat surface, covered over so they cannot be seen. Ask that the cover be lifted for 15 seconds. After the cover is replaced, immediately write down the names of as many of the objects as you remember seeing.

Test 2: Have a colleague or friend test your *hearing recognition* and memory. Ask that a colleague orally give you a list of 20 common items in rapid succession. Immediately thereafter, write down the names of as many of the objects as you remember hearing.

Test 3: Have a colleague or friend test your *feeling recognition* and memory. Ask that 20 common objects be placed on a flat surface, covered over so they cannot be seen. You reach under the cloth for 15 seconds and feel as many of the objects as you can. Immediately thereafter, write down the names of as many of the objects as you believe you identified solely by feeling.

> **Evaluation 1:** Which test did you pass with the highest score? In other words, do you seem to be primarily a visual learner, an oral learner, or a kinesthetic learner?

Test 4: A new friend wants to give you directions to get from your house to his, and it's going to take several miles and several turns.

1. Do you want him to give you a map so that as he describes where to turn and in which direction, you can follow his explanation by putting your finger onto the map, tracing the route as he tells you what to do? Or,
2. Do you want him to tell you how to go, after which you will ask him to listen as you repeat what he told you to get confirmation that you have memorized the turns correctly? Or,
3. Do you want to have a map in front of you while he's giving you the explanation so that you can see on the map what he's describing?

> **Evaluation 2:** Based on your answer to Test 4, are you primarily a kinesthetic, oral, or visual learner?

If you are a kinesthetic learner, you'll need to include decoding and phonics methods, along with the kinesthetic, to help your non-reader get started.

But if you are primarily a visual or oral learner, you are not to use either of these methods exclusively. You should, in fact, make sure that most of your instruction is kinesthetic.

And remember, what you are doing is remedial; that is, you are using a proven remedy to replace failure with success.

Step 1

Begin the New Learning Arrangement

WHAT EQUIPMENT DO YOU NEED?

Essential

- a sand tray made of flat plastic or metal sheet with sides deep enough to hold approximately one-half inch of sand
- a fat black crayon
- some strips of somewhat stiff white- or buff-colored paper, stiff enough to resist tearing when the student traces the crayon writing. The strips can be cut from an 8.5 x 11 inch piece of paper by folding the paper in half, then in half again so that each strip is about 2 inches wide and 11 inches long.
- a box to hold 3 x 5 inch index cards, a set of dividers indicating A, B, C, and so forth, and, of course, unlined index cards to be placed in the box
- some soft pencils and scrap paper
- a typewriter or computer hooked to a printer
- a three-hole notebook and three-hole unlined paper; you also may want stiff paper to be used for a cover and some brads to create a "book" of a story told by your pupil
- some library books, not "easy-to-read" beginning-reader

books, but a few books that pupils who can read, like to read; include some poetry, fiction, and nonfiction. You will need to know what interests your pupil. Which poems have special meaning? Which make-believe stories catch his or her imagination? Which facts have special meaning? Are cars or trucks or airplanes a special interest? What about tools? What about buildings? What about famous people? What about animals, or places like a volcano? It is you, the teacher, who will be doing the reading, so you can start with books that your pupil would have liked to learn to read.
- most of all, a place to do the teaching that is private and quiet and comfortable, even better if you can work at a table large enough for you both to sit there and have the sand tray handy and room for the strips of stiff paper, black crayon, soft pencil, and plenty of scratch paper. A blackboard (or equivalent) is very helpful. If there's not one on the wall, you can use a "slate"; that is, an individual writing surface easily erased.

Helpful

- some number and alphabet blocks—particularly the kind of squares made of wood or plastic that have raised letters and numerals
- a set of 10 individual numerals, 0–9, made of plastic or wood
- sets of identical-sized objects, like 20 plastic straws or 20 rubber erasers or 20 large paper clips or . . .

WHAT GUARANTEE DO YOU GIVE YOUR PUPIL?

Remember: Your pupil has failed for some three years and is probably scared that more failure lies ahead.

Start the lesson explaining that it's now up to you—the

teacher—to get it right. Guarantee that you will succeed, and your pupil will learn to read. You are not going to quit, and most importantly, you are going to blame yourself, not your pupil, if some lesson isn't successful.

NOW, THAT SAID, HOW SHOULD YOU BEGIN?

Ask your pupil what word he wants to learn. He says, "I don't know." You say, "I don't either; it's up to you to tell me the word and up to me to teach you how to write it and read it."

> **Caution:** The length of time for the initial lesson is enormously important and impossible to guess up front. You should not preset your time. I once stopped after six minutes with the pupil complaining he was ready for more teaching, but he was shaking with fear. We had managed for him to succeed writing the first letter of his first name, and he couldn't believe his good fortune. So, I reminded him that I was going to succeed as his teacher and that we would meet again the next day.

If you don't already know, ask your pupil whether he writes left- or right-handed. Important: Angle your writing that is to be traced to follow your pupil's natural style. If your pupil has been taught to print, then print and gradually move to cursive. If he is left-handed and slants the letters "backward," write the word that way.

I once was given the word "gorilla" by a new pupil. I panicked. One "r" or two? One "l" or two? I excused myself from our work table, looked it up in the dictionary, and came back ready to write the full word in the sand tray. Then I remembered to find out if he was left- or right-handed (right) and whether he wanted me to print the word or to use cursive (cursive).

I shook the tray and wrote "gorilla." As I wrote it, I strung out the sounding of the word. He watched closely. Then, with his right index finger, he traced over my writing of gorilla in the sand; he traced it again.

Next I took a strip of stiff buff-colored construction paper and with the fat black crayon wrote the word "gorilla" on the long side of the paper while I said the word. He traced over the letters with the index and middle fingers of his right hand and at the same time said the word. He actually got some of the black crayon on his fingers, as I intended.

We took a break. We took a drink. We went for a walk. We looked in a couple of dictionaries, and I found the right page showing both the word "gorilla" and a good drawing. He told me he had recently been to the zoo and seen a gorilla, and that's why he wanted to learn to write the word. Then we went back to our work table.

I wrote "gorilla" in the sand while saying the word, and he traced over my letters saying "gorilla." He shook the sand tray, and I wrote/spoke the word again; he traced my writing and said the word. He "erased" the sand tray.

I gave him the strip that I had already made, and that he had traced once before, and he traced over the black crayon writing again, saying the word.

I asked him if he was seeing the gorilla drawing in one of the dictionaries. "No, I'm thinking about the one I saw at the zoo; he smelled awful."

WHAT THRILLS YOU DURING A LESSON?

I was thrilled. This meant that he was not just moving his fingers and lips, but he was actually "feeling" the word as a "gorilla." He traced the crayon word several more times.

Next I asked that he write the word in the air. With him beside me so that our fingers would be moving in the same direction, we wrote "gorilla" as though we were tracing it. He started off strong on "go." And finished strong with "lla." So I asked him to trace the crayon-written word a couple more times.

Then we both did it in the air, and we came down hard on the sound "r."

I asked him to trace the crayon word one more time, then turn the paper over and write "gorilla" across the top of the narrow side with his soft pencil.

This student did it the first time, but if he had not, I would not have drawn his attention to what was incorrect; instead, I would have crossed the whole word out and asked him to turn the strip over and trace it again, looking at what he was doing and saying the word slowly as he did the tracing. When he had done it what he thought was enough times, I would have suggested that he turn the paper over again and write the word correctly below the one I had crossed out.

WHEN SHOULD YOU STOP THE FIRST TRACING LESSON?

Had the student failed the second time, I would have ended the writing portion of this first lesson.

Had he gotten it correct, I would have ended the writing portion of this first lesson.

In fact, as soon as he had "mastered" the word "gorilla," I would have stopped the writing portion of the lesson and given him free time to go to the bathroom, get a drink, have a snack, take a walk, or use playground equipment.

And then we would have had the reading portion of the lesson. His choice. This particular pupil, as requested, had brought with him to our tutoring session a storybook for the reading time, but when I asked him what he wanted to hear me read, he said he wanted me to read what the dictionary said about the gorilla.

Fortunately, the classroom had a set of encyclopedias, and after reading from the dictionary, we read from there about the gorilla as well.

He went home exhausted; his parents reported that he slept soundly for several hours when he got home.

SO, WHAT WILL YOU DO FOR YOUR FIRST LESSON?

Just about the same as I did for my pupil. The word your pupil chooses undoubtedly won't be the same, but the process will be: learning it first by tracing in the sand, then over black crayon, then in the air, and finally by writing it on the back of the crayon strip.

But wait! It may be that you don't get past the sand-tray tracing because your pupil is too anxious to concentrate, or unwilling to trace carefully, or unwilling to look at the word, or silent when asked to say the word.

In other words, his or her behavior may be abominable! Your pupil may not believe that it's you who are responsible for his learning to read. If he won't trace the letters in the sand, but just messes the sand, put the sand tray away.

Go to the black crayon and strip of construction paper, and then into the air.

If necessary, just place the first letter of the word on the construction paper and have him trace that letter, giving it the sound (hard or soft) that it has in his chosen word. Move to writing just that letter in the air.

Maybe stop the lesson after he learns this first letter. Offer to read aloud from his chosen book, and stop the lesson after less than 10 minutes.

Can you guess what you should do to start the second lesson with a pupil who has not learned the given word during the first lesson? Your answer is important!

Step 2

Jump into Lesson 2

HOW DO YOU START THE SECOND LESSON?

Your pupil did not learn the word she traced in the first lesson. How should you start this second lesson? Should you work on that word, or ask your pupil for a new word? Actually, it's not your decision!

Ask your pupil whether she wants to learn a new word, or whether she wants to continue working on learning the word from the first lesson. She's probably going to choose a new word, but what to do if she chooses the "old" word?

Treat the word like it's new. Don't refer to any work done previously. Start with the sand tray; then go to writing with the crayon. Be sure to test her learning in the air.

If it's still not coming easily, talk with your pupil about what's hard about it.

Never have your pupil trace only part of the word; always have her trace the whole word. Yet, you may want to talk about the difficulty of a silent letter or a combination of letters that are causing some of the difficulty.

Generally, the word you will be given by this nonreader is one that can be pictured: a name of a person or thing; a number; a month; a holiday; a favorite place or toy. Talk about the "picture" of the word, as I talked about the gorilla, and found pictures of gorillas, and heard from my pupil about the live gorilla he had seen and smelled in the zoo.

The more alive the word is to your pupil, the more reason she has to trace it and to reproduce it correctly.

Your pupil will not be thinking of how to learn 10,000 words if learning just one word takes at least two lessons! No, your pupil will only be thinking about whether you have told her the truth: that you can teach her to read and write a word she wants to know.

And you, the teacher, you should not be thinking that it will take years and years to teach your pupil even a basic 2,000 words if it takes two days to teach just one. What you must believe, and your pupil will discover, is that this is the best remedial teaching method for you to use, culminating in your pupil learning how to teach herself to read.

What should you do if your pupil apparently did learn the first word during the first lesson?

SHOULD YOU REVIEW?

Yes and no. Again, it is up to your pupil.

Ask your pupil whether she wants to review the last lesson's word or learn a new word. Let's posit that she asks to review. And let's further posit that she has trouble with the word.

Ask your pupil if she wants to write the word herself in the sand tray. She does it and makes a mistake. Shake the pan immediately, getting the wrong writing out of sight and thought, and ask if she wants to try again, by herself, or whether she would like you to write it so that she can trace it.

If, on her second try, she does it correctly, take out the crayon sheet and ask her to trace the word, reminding her to say it and look at it closely as her fingers press on the crayon while writing.

Before asking her to turn the crayon sheet over, have her write the word in the air, perhaps the two of you writing it side-by-side in the air. If you are sure of her fluency, have her retrace the crayon writing once more, turn the paper over, block out what she wrote there yesterday, and write the word. If correct, leave as is. If incorrect, be sure to cross it out and turn the paper over to show the correct crayon writing.

Have your pupil trace and sound the word again, then in the air, then on the chalkboard. And finally, when you both agree she knows it, have her do one "final" tracing over the crayon and, covering what was written on the back, have her write the word again. If correct, congratulations are in order, and emphasize that the congratulations are for both of you!

If it is incorrect, leave that word. In fact, it's time for recess. You should also suggest that you leave further tracing of that word, or a new one, for the next lesson.

Now, if your pupil wants to try once more and you believe she will succeed, then, yes, help her trace again both in sand and over crayon. But if you believe she won't be able to do it correctly—perhaps too anxious—make the decision with her to have recess, then a story, and then if the energy is there, to use the counting materials to create combinations of numbers. (See explanation for how to do this at end of this chapter.)

Of course, she may have truly learned her first word, remembering it from the first lesson, and when you invite her to write it, she may do it correctly, first in the sand, then in the air, and finally on the chalkboard. It is good for the pupil to feel success. You should be quite satisfied that she knows how to recognize the word and how to sound the word, understands the meaning of the word, and knows how to write the word.

HOW SHOULD YOU USE THE INDEX CARDS?

If you are satisfied that your student has truly learned her word, now is the time to begin using the card file, alphabet dividers, and blank index cards.

With your guidance, your pupil should do the following:

1. Decide which letter of the alphabet starts her word.
2. Write the word on one of the blank index cards.
3. Decide what she wants on the card. For example, my "gorilla" pupil wanted a picture of a gorilla, and we used tracing paper so that he could do the outline from the illustration in the dictionary; then we taped the tracing onto the card. Or your pupil might want to dictate to you what she wants written on the card about her word. For example, a girl I was teaching who wanted to learn her last name, asked me to write on her card, "This is my father's name and mine, too."
4. File the card behind the correct letter.

> The card file is going to be a tangible picture and repository of success—of words the pupil has learned to read, to write, to understand.

BUT WHAT IF YOUR PUPIL WANTS TO LEARN A BRAND NEW WORD?

Do as you did in the first lesson. Start with you writing the word in the sand, slowly saying the word as you write it. As she traces your writing, be sure she is both looking at the word in the sand and saying the word correctly.

Remember to allow your pupil to shake the sand tray and erase the word. Invite her—when she is ready—to write the word in the sand by herself. If done well, you write the word with fat black crayon on the strip of stiff paper. Say the word as you do it. Invite her to trace it with index and middle fingers, looking at the word and sounding it as she traces each letter. Then when you are both satisfied that she knows how to write the word, side-by-side, both of you write it in the air and sound it as you do.

> **Caution:** You want your pupil to sound the whole word s-l-o-w-l-y, but you never want her to sound letter by letter. It's quite all right to break the word into sound syllables, for example, "go-ril-la."

> A quick lesson in the separating of words by sound: Some current dictionaries use what is called a "morpheme boundary" to break words for printing purposes when type is justified. A simple way to explain that boundary is when your mouth changes shape in the pronunciation. Again, gorilla is split three ways, but the sounding might divide into "go-rill-a." One shape of mouth for "go," another for "rill," and a third for "a."

Remember: If your student knows only printing, for these first lessons you should print. But one of your aims is to move to cursive as soon as you can as the flow of the letters helps the flow of the sound.

WHEN IS QUITTING TIME?

It's entirely up to you how many words you want to introduce in lesson 2; not words you suggest, but words your pupil wants to learn. If sand tracing, crayon tracing, air writing, perhaps chalk writing, and finally correct writing of the word without looking at it begins to go fairly smoothly, you must stop the lesson before your pupil wants to stop!

That's important. Let me repeat: While the words you teach to your pupil are the pupil's to choose, quitting time is yours. And you want to stop the tracing/writing portion of each lesson—particularly during the first 10 or so lessons—while the pupil is still interested in doing the work.

WHEN DO YOU READ ALOUD?

Daily for early lessons, you will read from a book that appears particularly interesting to your pupil. Talk about what you are reading together, explain meanings of words, clarify use of certain words and phrases—make this reading-aloud portion of the tutoring session one that celebrates your pupil's native intelligence. Always do the reading after you've finished with the tracing of words and had a recess.

My "gorilla" pupil who wanted to have me read to him about gorillas during his first lesson and not from the storybook he had brought with him to the session also wanted to show me he could pick out the word "gorilla" in the dictionary and in the encyclopedia. But for our second lesson—after he delightedly demonstrated he could write "gorilla" correctly in the sand, in the air, on the back of the crayon paper, and on the index card—he asked that I start reading from the book he had brought with him.

WHEN CAN YOU START
DOING SOME MATH?

We are still in the second lesson. If you feel your pupil is under too much stress, you can end the session after your reading. But ideally, after the reading time and a few minutes of recess—some active movement for your pupil—you want to start teaching your pupil how to solve math-related word problems.

You need those plastic or wooden numerals out on the table. Ask your pupil to arrange them from nine down to zero, across the surface horizontally or down the surface vertically—it matters not. You simply want the sequence to be correct.

Then ask that the numerals be arranged from zero up to nine.

Ask her to use three of the numerals to create the largest possible number. It cannot be 999, since she has only one 9. Ask her to create the smallest possible number using three of the numerals. Talk about it together. If she gets either task incorrect, reason out why. Reason out, as well, why the final answer is correct.

You should provide whatever help is necessary as this may be, simple as it is, a brand new task.

Ask your student to choose one of the numerals to trace its written name, and put the other nine out of the way. Write her chosen numeral in the sand. Have your pupil concentrate on what that numeral looks like as a symbol and as a written word in the sand tray. Have her watch you write each one in the tray. She should trace the symbol first while saying its name. Then she should trace the word, repeating the name.

Do the same with the black crayon on the stiff paper: trace both the numeral and the word.

In the air, do the same.

Finally, on the back of the black crayon strip, have her write first the symbol and then the word.

If you are sure that she has learned this symbol and word correctly and that it is now part of her reading vocabulary, you can ask her to write both forms on an index card and put it in the box: most pupils will do zero first.

In the next 10 lessons, you will teach all 10 numerals. Remember: It's your job to teach them, and if it takes 20 lessons, be patient, be positive, and be assured that you do know how to teach!

Also remember, you ask the pupil which numeral she wants to learn next.

HOW SHOULD YOU CLOSE LESSON 2?

Take a short recess, and plan one final activity to close lesson 2.

Clear the surface. Put out the 20 items—the erasers, or straws, or paper clips, or small same-size blocks.

Talk about what a "half" is, and ask that the student put the 20 items in two equal piles. Talk about how many should be in each pile, and let her count them one by one, or by pulling two together, or however she works at it naturally. It's important for you to notice just how she determines that she has exactly the same number of items in each pile.

You need to use this session to learn how your pupil learns. And you are learning how to teach her how to learn.

This first session with the items, play around with the items to create relationships. Here are some suggestions, but use your own imagination. Keep in mind, though, you are establishing numerical relationships and helping your pupil to become more familiar with the value of numbers.

- Put just eight items in a pile. Ask your pupil to split the pile in half; then ask that each half pile be split in half; then ask that each of the four piles be split in half. Ask your pupil how soon she realized that there would be eight single items after dividing the original eight in half three times?
- Now, play around with halving only even piles of items. Talk about, before dividing, whether your pupil thinks that a pile of 12 items will divide down into 12 single items.
- Make a list of those even-number piles that do divide down into singles, and make another list of those that do not. Lead a discussion with your pupil about why she thinks this happens.
- Ask your pupil if she thinks a pile with an odd number (three, five, seven, nine, etc.) of items can be split in half enough times to become single items? Why not?
- Write the following word problem on the chalkboard. Then you

read it aloud to your pupil as many times as she asks. Together you explore the answers.

Mary is 12 and her brother Bob is 6.
Bob is now half as old as Mary.
Was Bob half as old as Mary when he was 5?
How old was Mary when Bob was 5?

Step 3

Tackle Lesson 3

SHOULD YOU START WITH NEW WORDS OR REVIEW?

You and your pupil have learned to trace words and numbers in a sand tray. Together you have started a file box of index cards to build vocabulary recognition. You have read aloud to your pupil, discussing the story and exploring the illustrations. You have begun doing some math using the sand tray and have used some objects to move and count on a table top. You have remembered to balance free play time with learning-to-read time.

And now you are ready to continue tracing, writing, reading, and filing and to begin creating original stories.

Always begin these early lessons by tracing "old" words that the pupil chooses. (Do this for the pupil, because he knows he has already learned them and will enjoy the feeling of success.) When your pupil does not seem to need such reinforcement, start with a new word. Be sure to start with you writing the word in the sand tray, and your pupil—with the index finger of his writing hand—tracing over the path you have made in the sand. You should say the word aloud as you write it; your pupil should say the word aloud as he traces it.

Do this until your pupil can write the word in the sand tray.

Next, sitting side-by-side, both of you write the word in the air.

Next, use a stiff piece of paper (one-quarter of an 8.5 x 11 inch sheet), stiff enough to resist tearing when the pupil traces the crayon writing. Say the word as you write it with a soft black crayon on the long side of the stiff paper. Your pupil should use the index and middle fingers of his writing hand and trace over the crayon wax while saying the word.

When both you and your pupil agree that he has learned the word, turn the paper over and have the pupil write the word from memory at the narrow end.

If successful, go on to another word.

If unsuccessful, you and the pupil decide whether you should go back to the sand tray or just retrace the crayon writing. But before you do, cross out the wrong spelling, or if you have opaque tape, put it over the mistake.

> A sight learner actually learns from looking at incorrect/correct spellings written side-by-side after being shown how to choose the correct one. This is not a helpful learning method for a kinesthetic learner.

You and your pupil should work on learning as many new words as your pupil wants to learn, but be alert to the ideal quitting time. Remember, you want to stop this part of the lesson while your pupil is still willing to continue and before you think his wavering concentration may turn into mistakes. Think about it: Your pupil has already spent three times 180 days in school failing to learn these same words! Do whatever you can to avoid another failure!

WHEN SHOULD YOU ADD TO THE FILE BOX?

When you are sure your pupil has "conquered" a word, have him write it on an index card and together decide what information or drawing to put on the card to provide one or more meanings for the word.

Also, invite your pupil to look at any other words now in the file box, reviewing them with you.

Important: Do not ask your pupil to spell one of the words in the file box orally. Instead, you might invite him to join you in writing the word in the air (sitting side-by-side) and next, if it seems appropriate, ask your pupil to write it on the chalkboard.

If the pupil makes a mistake, erase the whole word quickly. Invite him to look and say the word from the index card again. If you think it necessary, suggest that you write it in the sand and that your pupil trace it there, then in the air, then on the chalkboard.

As you do this review, praise each step.

Time for recess.

WILL YOU TELL ME A STORY?

Put away the sand tray, file box, crayons, and paper strips. Take a piece of scrap paper, or go to the typewriter or to the computer keyboard.

You are going to invite your pupil to tell you a short story. If you think it will help, you can tell your pupil about my pupil—the story I will now tell you.

When we got to this part of his lesson, my "gorilla" pupil dictated one sentence: "I saw a gorilla at the zoo."

I wrote that sentence first on a piece of scrap paper.

I asked him if he wanted to give his story a title.

"Yes. 'The Gorilla.'"

I took one of the sheets from the three-hole notebook and, using the typewriter, wrote in a large font his title, a line for the author, and, allowing some space, his sentence, that is, his "story."

I then invited him to read the story to me. He read what he remembered dictating: "I saw a gorilla at the zoo." I had to remind him to read the title. This he did, and reread both the title and the story sentence aloud.

Then I invited him to illustrate the story.

He did something quite clever. He drew a sign with a post stuck in the ground. And looking at my typed story, he wrote the word "zoo" on the sign with an arrow pointing ahead.

He had not asked to learn the word "zoo," in any of the three earlier lessons, so I asked him if he would like to trace it, learn it, and add it to the file box. He was eager to do this.

You need to do something similar with your pupil. Even if he wants to dictate a long story, convince him to do a short one for his first. You want him to remember what he dictated, so that when you have it printed on the three-hole notebook paper, he can "read" it aloud. That is, he can remember what he dictated.

After my pupil read the title of his story and the one sentence making up the story, we put that story in the three-hole notebook. After a brief second recess, he put the plastic (or wooden) numerals on the table.

WHEN IS IT TIME TO LEARN A SECOND NUMBER?

After this first story is written, it is time for your pupil to learn more numbers. Remember to let your pupil choose which number he wants to learn. Say he chooses seven. In the sand put the numeral (7) and the word (seven). Have your pupil trace the "7" asking him to think of how many objects that is; then trace the word, saying its name.

Next, sitting side-by-side with your pupil, write first the "7" and then "seven" in the air.

Next, use the crayon and stiff strip of paper. You write the numeral and the word; next your pupil gets his writing-hand finger dirty with black crayon tracing over your writing.

If it seems helpful, write both numeral and word with chalk, and have your student trace over the chalk.

Return to the crayon strip, and when he feels ready, turn the strip over and across the narrow end have your pupil write first the "7" and then "seven."

It is your pupil's choice: does he want to review the number he learned in lesson 2 by tracing it? If so, work together on that numeral and its word form until you both are sure your pupil knows how to both read it and write it.

Remove everything from the table but your 20 counting items, a pencil, and some scrap paper.

Place the 20 counting items on the table in a single pile, and ask your pupil to put 7 of them in a vertical line. Then put 7 of them in a horizontal line. Push the other 13 items out of the way, and then ask him how many ways he can divide the 7 items into two piles.

1 and 6
2 and 5
3 and 4

Suggest that the order could be reversed, so now place them like this:

6 and 1
5 and 2
4 and 3

Perhaps he has already stumbled onto yet another way, to have a place with no item and all seven in the other pile.

0 and 7
7 and 0

That should have been done orally as piles were divided. But now to a written record.

Again put the seven items into a pile, and after the separation into two piles, ask your pupil to write what he has done on a piece of scrap paper. For example, he might have put one item in one pile and six in the other. He should then write $1 + 6 = 7$.

I don't mean for you to dictate which combination should be written first. I do mean that after your pupil has made the separation of the seven items, while they are still in front of him, he should write the record of what he has done. It might be $0 + 7 = 7$ or $5 + 2 = 7$. But have your pupil do all eight of the combinations—first moving the items into piles, then stating orally each combination, then recording (as an equation) on scrap paper what has been done.

Do not let your pupil skip the moving of the items into the correct size piles.

Do not let him skip the stating orally of what he has done.

Before a second short recess, be sure that your pupil has learned his new number word, as well as the numeral. Perhaps ask him to write it in the sand tray after you write the numeral. Or do this on the blackboard. Or use the crayon strip. And when you are sure that the new number has been learned, have your pupil write both the numeral and the word on an index card. Have your pupil show seven objects (or how many the numeral and its written name means) on the index card. Use the back if needed.

HOW DO YOU TEACH MORE NUMBER RELATIONSHIPS?

First, ask your pupil to

1. put 12 of the items in one pile.
2. split that pile in half; ask how many in each half.
3. split one pile of 6 in half; ask how many in each half.
4. put the 12 items back into one pile.
5. divide the 12 items into three piles with the same number in each pile.

6. determine how many there are in each third.
7. put the 12 items back into one pile.

Then, explain that you are going to ask that the items be divided into four piles, but before your pupil does this, he is to guess whether there will be the same number in each pile as there were in each of the three piles, fewer than in each of the three piles, or more than in each of the three piles. On scrap paper, you write his choice:

Just the same number?
Fewer?
More?

Now have your pupil divide the 12 items into the four equal piles and check whether his guess was correct.

At this point, invite your pupil to do some dividing of the 12 items, telling you what he is doing. As soon as he divides them, talk about the pattern he has made and help him record the pattern either on the chalkboard or on the scrap paper—just the numerals, not the words.

Let's say, for example, he puts one item in one pile, two in another, three in another, four in the next, and two in the last. Help him to write $1 + 2 + 3 + 4 + 2 = 12$. Or he may make piles that show $1 + 2 + 3 + 3 + 2 + 1 = 12$.

Step 6, "Season with Mathematics throughout the Lessons," has scores of similar activities for you to use.

Notice, you are using the kinesthetic learning method with the touching and moving of the items. You are using the oral method by having your pupil articulate what he is doing while moving the items. And you are using the visual method by having your pupil watch what he is doing, writing it down and making a "picture" of what he has done with the items. In this way, you are helping him to prove to himself that he has the ability to read what he has written. Not just to read it, but to understand the meaning of what he is reading.

WHEN IS IT STORY TIME?

Of course, after the math work, take a short recess, and end this third lesson by reading aloud a story your pupil wants to hear.

This does not need to be a different story every day, but your pupil well may have chosen a really interesting storybook with many chapters. Or, he really may wish to hear a story a second time or even a third time. It is your pupil's choice!

Whether it is a new story, an old story, or more of a long story, be sure each day to review orally what happened during the previous reading(s). If you are not in agreement about something that was said or done, be sure to find the place and read aloud a clarification.

Don't make this review boring; get on with the story if it is taking several readings. And if it is a brand new story, only briefly review the previous one. If the pupil hasn't chosen a story that he actually wants to hear, be sure to invite him to choose another. You might have a book of poems on hand to read from if the book the pupil has brought turns out not to be to his liking.

Choose poems with good humor and that create interesting mental pictures.

What Should Be Included in Each Lesson Period?

This third lesson, and the next 50 or 100, most often should consist of these several elements:

1. Tracing new words
2. Adding new words to the file box
3. Dictating and reading a story
4. Doing and recording some math
5. Listening to a story

Step 4

Take Stock

> Dear Tutor:
> Please reread steps 1, 2, and 3. As you read them, think about how your pupil has done on all the teaching you have provided.
> Please reread the foreword, by Mark Perkins, head of The Forman School. He explains that every student is different; "not all students are 'wired' to pick up reading naturally." He further explains the need for a "comprehensive plan to guarantee your student's success." Is the way you are teaching comprehensive enough?
> This really is a recipe book, and you may need to scrap a dish or two that didn't work out. Never mind. You can teach the work again, this time making particularly sure you are following the recipe meticulously.
> I can assure you that I have done an enormous amount of re-writing, re-thinking, re-wording, and, yes, praying that what you read here will turn into, for you, successful teaching.
>
> Sincerely,
> *Cynthia Parsons*

WHAT SHOULD YOU DO AFTER THE 20TH LESSON TRACING NEW WORDS?

This is a key decision. Do you still need to have your pupil use the sand tray? Or perhaps you need to

- write each new word with black crayon on a stiff piece of paper.

- have your pupil trace over it, saying the word, while looking at the word.
- discuss the meaning and use of the word.
- trace the word in the air, both of you, sitting side-by-side.
- have the pupil again trace over the black crayon until she is sure she knows how to write the word.
- have the pupil turn the stiff piece of paper over and write the word from memory across the narrow end with a soft pencil. Turn the strip of paper over and check whether what the pupil wrote is correct. If incorrect, you cross it out, and have the pupil trace it again both on the strip of paper and in the air. And when you are satisfied she knows how to spell the word, turn the strip of paper over and have your pupil write it from memory.

> **Remember:** You can call "quitting time" if you feel it best. Do not, do not let your pupil fail more than once. Perhaps it would be good to use the sand tray for a while longer.

Is the sand tray still an excellent way to have your pupil focus entirely on the desired outcome—learning to read, write, spell, and understand the meaning of a new word? Instead of using first the crayon version, you might first write the word yourself in the sand tray, shake, and then have your pupil write it there.

Whether or not you use the sand tray for subsequent lessons, do not abandon writing in the air, or crayon tracing, or pencil writing on the back side of the crayon strip.

Surely by the 20th lesson, you should be using cursive and not manuscript printing. Start with shorter words—"dog," for example. You might want to show the manuscript printing of a word on the chalkboard, but use cursive in the sand tray and with the black crayon.

After tracing the cursive, you might invite your pupil to show you how the same word can be printed. Be sure your pupil understands that the difference is penmanship and not spelling or meaning!

Surely by the 20th lesson, you should be exploring the meanings of each word, sharing together when there are several meanings and thinking of ways to distinguish them. For example, I was working with a fourth grader, and he chose the word "pin." I asked him the meaning, and he responded, "Two points."

He said it with such authority that I had enough sense to ask for a clarifying sentence instead of suggesting he was wrong. His brief sentence was "Two points for a pin." "Ah," I said, "wrestling."

But we went further; we discussed "pinning" someone down while wrestling with ideas instead of bodies. Then, proving he seriously understood this word, he said, "When you and my dad talk, you are always pinning!"

We also discussed safety pins and blanket pins (he was a farm boy), and straight pins, and diaper pins, and Velcro!

"Pin" is a wonderful word for a kinetic learner! Like "ball," it comes in a wonderful variety easy to picture and easy to think of handling.

Then he asked, "Can I put pin and pins and pinning on my card?" If he had not asked, I would have asked him if he wanted to add these new words to his index file. I would have given him the option to put all three words—"pin," "pins," and "pinning"—on one card, or to make one card for the nouns and one for the verbs.

I asked if he wanted to trace pins and pinning in the sand tray, and he said he would rather just do it on the crayon strips. That was our last lesson using the sand tray. I kept it handy and sometimes used it for math, but he was ready to learn new words by going from crayon to air to chalk, back to crayon, and finally to the index card.

WHAT ABOUT USING "PIN" FOR SOME PHONICS?

Yes and no.

You must gauge the moment for this. A good way to teach the similar sounds is to place a learned word, such as "pin," on the chalkboard. Ask your pupil to suggest another three-letter word that sounds like pin.

Let's assume her first response is "win." Before asking your pupil to write it on the chalkboard, talk about what it means. Then ask what letter she thinks it starts with. If she knows it is "w," let her write the correct letter on the chalkboard. If there is some hesitancy, write the letter with the black crayon on a strip. Have your pupil trace the letter, then turn the strip over and have her write it across the top correctly; then invite her to write "win" on the chalkboard.

And so with other words she suggests. Suppose she says "thin." Explain that it has four letters, and we want only three this time. "Tin" may come, but probably not "bin" or "sin." "Fin," especially if fishing is a known activity, may be her choice. It might take some explaining to add "kin" to the list.

No need to exhaust the possibilities. Best for you to call quitting time while there is still interest in learning how to spell words that "sound" so similar to pin and end in "-in." Also best to start with three-letter words, since for your kinesthetic learner, oral/aural learning may be secondary or even third behind look-see.

This is a grand way to add words to the card file and a good time to review some or all of the cards.

But let us consider the question again. Is it time for you to begin giving your pupil phonics lessons? If you put "pin" on the chalkboard and ask for another three-letter word sounding the same and your pupil seems confused, just suggest one example, explore its meaning, allow her to trace it, and add it to the index box—but wait until a later lesson to begin developing learning some words by hearing and repeating sounds.

Both the "in" sound and the "at" sound—as in "hat," "fat," "sat," "cat," and so on—are good starters to develop good listening skills. Remember: Your pupil failed to learn when she had phonics lessons for the first three years in school. You want to be sure she knows the first word well enough that sounding and "seeing" similar words now comes easily.

Hence, use caution. Be sure there is an opportunity for your pupil to trace each sounded word once, either in the sand or over the crayon writing. Be sure she has an opportunity to write each word in the air. Be sure each word is written on the chalkboard. Then after the kinesthetic lessons, it's safe to add "sounded" words to the index box.

The time to start learning four-letter words in a phonics lesson is when your pupil begins asking for them during the tracing period. Let's assume your pupil has reason to want to learn the word "thin," and either on her own or with a hint from you, she realizes this has the sound of "pin."

"Thin," "twin," "skin," and so on can be shown to sound and look like "pin." But do not teach this as an oral lesson. In a single row on the chalkboard, write a list of the three-letter "-in" words your pupil has learned in a prior lesson, and in a second row begin putting some four-letter "-in" words that your pupil suggests. But do not put the new four-letter "-in" words on the board until your pupil has traced them.

You want your pupil first to feel the word, then to see the word while hearing it.

Just to make sure you understand—if your pupil has asked to add "skin" to the list, you first have your pupil learn how to write the word "skin" by tracing the word "skin."

Yes, to anticipate your next question: There will come a time when tracing will no longer be necessary, but never a time when writing will not be.

HOW CAN YOU USE THE DICTATED STORY TO LEARN NEW WORDS?

For at least the first 10 lessons, encourage your pupil to dictate short stories to you, just a few sentences in each. Your main purpose, at first, is for your student to be able to read her own story with little or no help from you. "I saw a gorilla at the zoo." When faced with this "story" after an absence of a day or more, your pupil may need some prompting.

And you probably are well aware that the word "saw" may prove difficult for your pupil to read. Children who aren't reading by the end of the third grade tend to "see" letters in reverse order. In this way, "saw" becomes "was"; hence the power of tracing the word while saying the word.

For the first 10 or so dictated stories, you just want to help your pupil decide on an illustration and delight in reading the story back to your pupil after she has read the story to you.

You want to make thorough use of your pupil's stories to teach her how to read. This is what I did with "The Gorilla." I retyped it. I made a list of the words in the story below the text in the order they came in the story. Like this:

The Gorilla
I saw a gorilla at the zoo.

I
saw
a
gorilla
at
the
zoo

Remember: We did not trace all the words in that story the first day. We only traced "gorilla" and "zoo." Therefore, I asked the pupil to look in his index box to find out whether we had the words "saw," "a," "at," and "the" already in the box. We traced any new words starting with the sandbox. He wanted to check on "gorilla" and "zoo" at the same time.

The next day, I re-typed the story, and this time made an alphabetical listing of the individual words in the story:

a
at
gorilla
I
saw
the
zoo

I then asked him to start with the title and to read just the story. Then I held an index card over the lower words and one by one asked him to read each word. If he hesitated, I asked him to find the word in the story (which I had not covered up), then look below at the single word to help remember what it said.

You may be surprised that when your pupil is asked to tell you the word "the" sitting alone outside any context, she may not remember what it is; turning back to its use in the story gives it meaning. This is especially true during the first 20 or 30 lessons.

Is your pupil going to have trouble reading the words she has dictated in her story the first time you show them to her out of context? Yes, undoubtedly. That is why it is good to start with short stories at the beginning and to make both lists: first the words in the order they come in the story and then, on a separate day, the words in alphabetical order.

With successful tracing, these words may be written by the pupil on the index cards and filed behind the first letter.

When the story gets longer, list only new words, first as they appear in the story and later in alphabetical order. Enlist your pupil's help looking in the file box to see whether a word is already there. Actually, try to make the file box your pupil's domain. When something needs to be looked up, let the pupil do it. When something needs to be added, have your pupil do that activity.

Of course, the file box will disappear in favor of a good dictionary, but that step won't come at or near the 20th lesson. And the move should be made by the pupil. I have had pupils throw the card files away. I have had pupils save the files. It's up to your pupil, not you!

WHEN AND HOW DO YOU CREATE A BOOK FROM THE STORIES?

You create a book when your pupil really wants to do this.

Two personal experiences illustrate the answers to these questions.

One of my pupils, aged 10, used the same theme in several stories. He loved model cars, had several, and his stories were filled with their activities—both possible and imaginary.

The moment I asked him if he would like me to type some of the stories on fresh paper (without the lists of words) so that he could make them into a book, he was quick to explain that we should do the book for the four-year-old brother of a friend. *Cars for Buddy* was the result.

I used good-quality blank three-hole paper and a large and very readable font. The pupil chose three of his stories, and when he had the new typed versions, he began illustrating the pages with cars and parts of cars.

He chose the construction paper for the cover and printed on the cover with dark crayon, listing himself as both author and illustrator. (Yes, both words had to be traced and added to the index box.)

When the book was completed—by putting brads through the holes—I asked him to practice reading the book aloud by reading it aloud to me. He looked startled, so I quickly asked, "Would you like me to read it to you once?" This I did.

He read his book to me twice, his choice, and off it went with him at the end of the lesson.

A quiet word to his parents, and he was given the opportunity to read the book to his parents, to his grandparents, to an aunt, and to four-year-old Buddy, and then he placed it on the bookcase in his own bedroom where it stayed for a long time—long after he had written several other books.

Another pupil wrote several imaginary stories about a girl who hated her teacher. She wanted to make a book of these stories and explained it was for her parents. I helped her just as I had helped the boy with the car stories. It was a test for me. I did everything I knew as a teacher to pass her test.

After she read the book to me, she put it in her pack and supposedly took it home. Her parents never mentioned it. I never saw it again. Her next book was made up of one long imaginary story full of curious animals. She even wrote a poem that she later set to music. I do not read music, so I enlisted the help of a teacher who did, and together they created an original tune. Her parents arranged for her to go to a daycare center to both read the story and sing the song while playing it on the piano.

It was after that performance that her desire to trace and learn went into high gear.

You want your pupil to have an audience for each story. You are not enough! You are "just" the tutor. When I have more than one pupil working with me, I overlap their arrival/departure times so that they can read their stories to each other. They love doing this.

Reading either to a much younger child or to an elderly person is also excellent.

Step 5 will go into more depth about ways to use your pupil's own stories to help teach her to read more fluently.

WHAT KIND OF EXPLORATORY MATH SHOULD YOU BE TEACHING YOUR PUPIL?

You will need a copy of this year's almanac, a source I favor because it has so many statistics covering a wide range of subjects and is organized in such a way to make it easy for a child still learning to read. I lean toward *The New York Times Almanac*. What you are doing is helping your pupil learn how to make wise use of a good resource, and at the same time, you are providing him with an opportunity to use math to solve a problem.

> **Puzzle 1:** Which is higher, Mt. McKinley in the United States or Mt. Popocatepetl in Mexico?

You will need to assist your pupil to find the answer to which mountain is higher:

1. Write the word "mountain" in the sand tray.
2. Have your pupil trace "mountain" in the sand tray.
3. Discuss what letter the word begins with.
4. Look in the almanac index for the word "mountain."
5. Find the page that tells about Mt. McKinley and Mt. Popocatepetl.
6. Note the heights and subtract the difference.

After each exploration to find an answer, your pupil will become more familiar with the organization of the almanac and relish discovering that she can read well enough to find out what she wants to know.

> **Puzzle 2:** What is the greatest known depth in the Pacific Ocean?

1. Assist by writing the word "ocean" in the sand tray and then have your pupil trace it.
2. Keep it there so as you look together in the index, your pupil can follow each letter until the word he wants is "duplicated."

> **Puzzle 3:** What was the highest batting average for Ty Cobb? And what was the highest batting average for Ted Williams?

This is a difficult one, requiring the student to find several words on the way. Try these steps:

1. Start, of course, with "baseball"; sandbox and trace.
2. Next, teach "batting"; again, sandbox and trace.
3. Next, teach "Ty Cobb"; sandbox and trace.
4. Once you get to Ty Cobb, your pupil will have to find his highest batting average among 12 of the given numbers.
5. Next, teach "Ted Williams"; sandbox and trace. Then your pupil must search the six given numbers to find the largest.
6. Finally, of course, subtraction is necessary to decide not only which one—Ty Cobb or Ted Williams—has the highest batting average, but also how much higher than the other.

Explore the almanac, find references to words your pupil has already added to her file box, and make up questions. Then ask your pupil to browse in a section of some interest and ask you questions. At first, you will have to do most of the reading, but once your pupil begins looking at data related to a specific subject of interest to her, together you can devise questions requiring math functions with interesting answers. And your pupil will become familiar both with the words and with how to use the almanac as a reference tool.

It's good, too, to play a bit with numbers. Have your pupil divide 12 of the counting items into four piles of 3 items in each. Now, talk about adding, subtracting, multiplying, and dividing. Put the symbols you want your pupil to use, including equals (=) on the chalkboard. Use scrap paper to record what you do with the counting items.

Puzzle 4: What's three times three plus three plus three?

1. Teach your pupil to write this on the chalkboard thusly: (3 × 3) + (3 + 3) = ? As you say the sentence, have your pupil "translate" the words into the math symbols.
2. Before writing the answer, have your pupil use the four piles of three counting items.
   a. First put three of the piles in one pile and add them up. Record this as 3 × 3 = 9.
   b. Then put two piles of three counting items and add them, and record this as 3 + 3 = 6. If necessary, have the pupil use the extra counting items to make two piles, one of 9 and one of six, and count them together.
3. Celebrate your success.

Puzzle 5: How can you make 10 with four 3s?

1. Let your pupil fuss about with this question using her counting items.
2. After a brief time, write on the chalkboard (3 × 3) + (3 ÷ 3) = 10. You may need to have a good discussion about why any number divided by itself is "1," and this is a good vehicle for your pupil to understand this.

Does your pupil understand that a fraction is a divided number? After asking a few more questions about what numbers can be found by using four 3s and only four 3s, invite your pupil to make one up.

Be sure to have your pupil record every activity on the chalkboard as well as on scrap paper. Be sure to ask her to talk out what has happened. For example, she might say, "I multiplied three times three to get nine, then made the fraction three-thirds to get one more, and so my four 3s equal 10."

When she states the answer, be sure that she points to the items on the chalkboard and touches each one, reinforcing what she has written in numerals with what she is saying.

After some good familiarity with using four 3s, work together to count from zero to 10 using four 3s and only four 3s. A couple of the answers are not easy to come by, but the first few are easy.

For example,

$0 = (3 + 3) - (3 + 3)$, or
$0 = (3 \times 3) - (3 \times 3)$, or
$0 = (3 \div 3) - (3 \div 3)$, or yet another,
$0 = 33 - 33$

And 10 equals three-thirds plus three times three: $(3 \div 3) + (3 \times 3)$.

Step 6 will give more suggestions for ways to use math exploration. This work is especially important since your pupil needs to be able to carry out activities that both stimulate and reinforce her understanding that she is of normal intelligence. Remember, it has been a long three-year struggle for your pupil trying to learn what her classmates have learned and she has not.

What fun, then, for your pupil to do some math that's sophisticated enough to be interesting; what joy to succeed. And learning to read and write numbers comes more easily when their functions make sense.

What if your pupil uses four 3s and ends up with a negative number? For example, what if she writes $(3 + 3) - (3 \times 3) = ?$ Excellent! Don't only use positive numbers, but use negative ones as well.

Put the three plus three counting items in one pile, and after your pupil has removed (that's what minus does!) all that are there, have her count out how many more should have been there to take nine from six.

You surely could make it clear if you told her that she owed her dad nine dollars and gave him only six dollars, and then asked your pupil how many more dollars she needed to pay off her debt.

Stay with those four 3s for several lessons. They really help the thinking process!

Step 6 is full of good math explorations for the kinetic learner.

SHOULD YOU STILL BE READING ALOUD TO YOUR PUPIL?

Yes. Step 8 discusses when and why to stop reading.

Suffice it to say at this point in your pupil's tutoring, the more compelling the reading material the better. If your pupil doesn't know what she wants you to read, be sure that what you choose really interests her.

Ideally, after 10 or so lessons working with a new pupil, you should know her well enough to be able to choose reading material of compelling interest to her.

If you start a story and she clearly loses interest, drop it. Even if she has chosen the story, but finds as you read it that her choice was a mistake, no need to continue. Together choose something she really would like to hear.

Step 5

Dictate a Story

WHEN IS IT WISE TO STOP USING THE SAND TRAY?

For 999 of 1,000 pupils, it's easier to trace a new word on a flat surface than on a vertical chalkboard. Hence, some tracing should continue for many lessons, both in the sand tray and with the black crayon, gradually dropping the use of the sand tray.

Just as you are in charge of "quitting time," in each lesson for each activity, you need to be the one to stop the use of tracing in the sand tray. It would be better for you to have your pupil continue using the sand tray for a longer—rather than a shorter—time.

It's akin to the use of the 20 counting items. There will come a time when your pupil won't need to move x number of rubber erasers into x numbers of piles in order to determine their value, but will be able to "image" them in thought.

If your pupil readily thinks of three items added to three items as six items, it would be counterproductive to insist that he manipulate the items. But it is always good for him to write down what his thoughts are. In a sense, he is dictating to himself; remember, he's a kinesthetic learner.

This is why tracing over the black crayon, followed by tracing in the air, followed by writing the traced word across the top on the reverse side of the crayon tracing should continue until your pupil no longer needs to start learning a new word by tracing it.

There is also a "quitting time" for the card file. A dictionary has all the words your pupil needs. And you will find that as his reading skills progress, he turns to the dictionary for new words, and then may wish to copy them onto an index card, proud to be building his own supply of words. Don't stop him from doing this. Let the "quitting time" come naturally.

It's very tempting for you—the teacher—to suggest to your pupil which words he might want to learn during the first portion of your lesson time. Resist that temptation! You get to suggest words when you work with him when he is reading the story he dictated. You get to suggest words when you are doing math together.

It's most important that your pupil initiate the words he wants to learn by tracing. After all, it is your pupil who is going to have to learn new words without tracing them. It is your pupil who has to teach himself how to use what he sees and what he sounds, and he needs to reproduce the words he wants to use as both a reader and a writer.

To remember words and numbers, your pupil needs to write them down. Eventually, the writing itself will be sufficient. A kinesthetic learner, for example, might write out a list of grocery items to purchase and mistakenly leave the list at home. When he gets to the store and discovers his mistake, he may be able to "feel" what he wrote earlier and hence fulfill his exact list. The writing was the only needed memory clue.

The visual learner, making the same mistake, won't "feel" what he wrote, but may be able to "see" what he wrote. And the oral learner, particularly if he sounded the names of the items while creating the shopping list, will be able to "hear" the missing items. All of us, of course, wish we had remembered to bring the list with us!

HOW CAN YOU MAKE EXCELLENT USE OF THE DICTATED STORY?

After the first 20 or so lessons, encourage your pupil to dictate longer and longer stories. It is his choice whether they are fiction or nonfiction or a combination.

When you type your pupil's story, make proper paragraphing and punctuate correctly.

After you have had your pupil do his first reading of his story aloud to you, talk about why you put the paragraphs where you did and get agreement on the punctuation.

If your pupil dictates a poem (be sure to invite this activity), type a "first draft," discussing how your pupil wants the lines to go, and then do a final copy that reflects his wishes.

One of my pupils asked me to read from the poem "Hiawatha," by Henry Wadsworth Longfellow. She wanted to write a poem that not only was about Hiawatha but also used the same type of phrasing as Longfellow had. So, when I did the typing after the dictation, I followed Longfellow's lead. This particular pupil dictated her poem about Hiawatha day after day and asked for Longfellow's "Hiawatha" for all reading sessions. Interestingly, during the early tracing lessons, she asked for what she called the "little common" words: "and," "for," "it," "to," "be," "but," "was," "is," "some," "today," and so forth.

She illustrated her Hiawatha poem by doing her drawings in a circle around the text. When she completed her book—if I remember correctly, it was more than 20 pages—she made a cover for it, put brads through the holes, and at the invitation of a daycare center, went there several days and read portions aloud to the children. She skillfully held the book up to show the illustrations and had the children look through the book with her while she talked about the illustrations.

Perhaps you can imagine what a thrill this would be for a pupil who had failed to learn to read day after day, week after week, year after year—to realize that now she could not only write and illustrate her own book, but also read it aloud to an appreciative audience without adult help!

Your pupil needs the same success—needs to make a book of whatever size, and needs to illustrate it and read it to an appreciative audience.

> **Caution:** Make sure you have an appreciative audience before allowing your pupil to read his book aloud. I had a lad with a wonderful imagination whose stories were science fiction and fantasy. His father, an engineer by training, had been hard on the boy for not learning to read at the rate he had as a child.
>
> When the youngster read his first dictated story to his father, it almost stopped our progress cold. The father was openly disdainful of his son's effort. I saw that we would have to keep the boy's work at the school and bring younger children and grandparents to the room to be the appreciative audience. Generally, most parents may even be more eager than the child to solve the "nonreader" problem and are eager to learn about each of the faltering first steps.

ARE YOU THE BEST AUDIENCE FOR YOUR PUPIL'S STORY READING?

This next statement may come as a surprise to you. The pupil you are tutoring will not consider you the "right" audience to listen to him read his story. This is very, very important.

You are the vehicle to make this glorious opportunity possible. Your role is key to the accomplishment. But, someone else, who wasn't part of the difficult learning period, is the right audience. You need to be humble about your teaching. The pupil will be grateful to you, make no mistake about that, but he probably will never refer to the role you played after he has become successfully literate.

One or both parents may always sing your praises. But for your pupil, the transition from loss to gain is a tender, difficult, and best-left-behind time.

I had a student who was severely disabled and who gained reading and writing skills that sent him successfully to college. Years later we met and he said, "I remember you were my tutor for a time, and that you read *20,000 Leagues under the Sea* to me. I really liked that book." He did not mention anything else about our lessons. Why?

He didn't want to be reminded of his "awful" failure to learn to read during those tortuous years in elementary school. He didn't want to be reminded of what kind of tutoring it required to bring him success in reading. He wanted a relationship with me that celebrated his interest in books, not one based on his earlier failures learning to read.

Fortunately, I had learned about this relationship from three superb remedial reading teachers at a small school in the San Jacinto Mountains of California. These teachers had each taught scores of children to read using a kinesthetic method. And they hovered over me during my first four years of teaching.

If you are a relative, particularly a parent or guardian, and you are the tutor, remember what you just read. Be very sensitive to your child's need for privacy.

WHICH WORDS SHOULD YOUR PUPIL TRACE FROM HIS DICTATED STORY?

As your pupil begins dictating longer stories, pick out the words you think he needs to trace in order to learn. On Tuesday, present Monday's story all typed, and list all the words in the story in the order in which they appear. Present duplicated words the first time only. On Wednesday, present Monday's story with just a few key words in alphabetical order. All these words are to be traced, recorded on index cards, and placed in the file box.

Here, I present a possible story and the word list for Tuesday:

My Smart Dog

My dog is really smart. If I throw a rubber ball, he will chase it. Then he will pick it up and put it in his mouth. When I call his name and say, "Come Buddy," he will bring me the ball. I have to take it out of his mouth and it is all wet.

The End

I want him to trace and learn the following words: smart, throw, rubber, chase, mouth, wet.

I would, though, put them in a column below the story in alphabetical order:

> chase
> mouth
> rubber
> smart
> throw
> wet

Why in this order? Why not in the order the words appear in the story? You want your pupil to have to read the word, not just remember it from the context of the story. "Wet," of course, would be a good word to use for some phonics practice. Remember, let your pupil choose the three-letter words spelled like "wet," only with a different first letter.

Is your pupil beginning to use the dictionary? Start with "a." Is there an "aet"? Go to "b," and locate "bet." Next, find "get." And so on. Should you use "debt"? No, your learner is kinesthetic; the learner who would love to include this four-letter word sounding like a three-letter word is a visual learner. If your dictionary includes the abbreviation "det," you will need to explain why an abbreviation is not a regular word.

Ah! But you can be clever. You can discuss why you are not including "debt." Maybe your pupil will ask for that word during the tracing lesson. Maybe your pupil will include it in the next story. Maybe he will just remember how it is different.

Of course, when you prepare one of the stories to be made into a book, you should not have the lists of words attached.

WHAT ABOUT THE PUPIL WRITING THE STORY ON A COMPUTER?

This is, of course, a positive progressive step.

You might start by having the pupil learn those six words in his smart dog story. After he has done so successfully, you retype the story until you get to one of those words, and you then invite your pupil to type the word he wants in there. Wonderful thing about the computer; it works like the sand tray—you can remove a mistake in a flash.

For example, your pupil wants to put in the word "smart." He gets the "s" and "m" correct and next puts in an "o." You call out, "Backspace!" Ask him to look in his card file, then finish the word.

In this case, six words typed by your pupil may be just the right number. You don't want to have him make mistakes, and you want to choose words that have so much meaning in the story that he will recall them.

Again, you are in charge of "quitting time" for the dictating of your pupil's stories. Eventually, you want your pupil to write his own story. You will provide spelling for every requested word. You will treat what he's written by hand in cursive script as a draft and help him to place punctuation correctly. And you will continue to type the story, type the lists of words he is to learn by tracing, and help him add those words to the file box. Then you will retype the story and your student will add his illustrations so that the story is suitable to be read aloud and shared with appreciative listeners.

WHAT IS A STRANGE AND WONDERFUL READING-ALOUD BOOK?

I had a pupil quite willing to do the tracing, work on the file cards, dictate a story, and do the math, but he was quite unwilling to listen to me read a story. He wouldn't bring a book for me to read and wouldn't want to listen to a story I chose.

His first name began with the letter "D." He liked writing that letter in all types of scripts. And that gave me an idea, one that worked not only for him, but for scores of other youngsters I've tutored.

I bought an incomplete set of an encyclopedia written for school children. Fortunately, the volume containing all "D" information was complete. I presented it to him as a gift and told him that at the close of each session, I would read anything in the volume he wanted and that in between he could take the book home.

He was thrilled. His own encyclopedia!

His dictation the very next day was based on something he had puzzled out for himself in his encyclopedia. His dictation every day thereafter came from things he was learning from his book. Every day I was told which part of the book to read aloud.

Where can you get, for next to nothing, an incomplete set of encyclopedias? Often public libraries have odd volumes they are happy to give away or sell for a pittance. And a lot of garage and lawn sales and even auctions of household goods have odd volumes of an encyclopedia for which the seller is delighted to get "anything." And I haven't yet met a child who wasn't thrilled to have his own initial!

WHAT ABOUT GIVING YOUR PUPIL A READING TEST?

You surely recall that it is you who is being tested, not your pupil. It is you who has given your pupil the guarantee that he will learn to read because of your appropriate teaching method.

Test yourself continuously:

- How is the tracing coming along? How few tracings are necessary today, and is that number less than yesterday's?
- Are the dictated stories getting more interesting, the vocabulary more mature, the sentence structure more complex?
- Can you see progress in your pupil's ability to explore math concepts? Is he grappling with more and more complex word problems?
- Are you finding the right problems that are not too easy to bother with nor too hard to try?

I was once part of a group teaching teachers (50 of them) how to teach elementary math in an exploratory manner. We took turns teaching a group of 10 students in the fifth grade. The director of our group complained that one of the students, Tony, wasn't participating, and hence we should excuse him from the class. It seems that several of the 50 teachers also wondered why Tony wasn't participating.

I liked Tony. He came early and helped me set up the recording equipment, so I asked him the next morning why he didn't speak up more when one of us was teaching. He said, "You never ask nothin' I don't already know."

Ah, he had it in an ungrammatical nutshell. I told the director, who, when it was his turn to lead the class, asked a question requiring a negative number as the correct response. All of the class was silent. Tony sat up straight, pointed his finger at the director and asked, "Can you go below?"

"What if you could?" countered the director.

"Then it's five, but not five that you have; it's five you don't have." And off the class went on negative numbers. It was the teacher who had to get the question right if he wanted the correct answer.

And this is your test. Every child of normal intelligence can learn to read. Some of them need a teacher to show the way. For your pupil, you are that teacher.

Step 6

Season with Mathematics throughout the Lessons

This is the longest step in this recipe book. Both steps 6 and 7 are full of resource information. Be sure to browse through these chapters frequently, looking for ways to make your tutoring sessions both more interesting and more effective.

For your pupil, some of the math explorations may be totally uninteresting: like six ways to cook broccoli in a cookbook for children. Others may trigger a very positive response. By the 10th tutoring session, you will probably know just which of the activities in this chapter will help your pupil be a better reader and mathematician.

WHAT MATH TERMS SHOULD YOUR PUPIL TRACE?

There are certain terms that will help your pupil understand and solve word problems. After tracing each of the following words and their appropriate symbols, have your pupil put the word and the symbol, perhaps several variations, on an index card. The symbols can, of course, be found in a dictionary or a junior high school math book.

Polygon = a closed two-dimensional figure with three or more sides
Area = the amount of space inside a polygon
Perimeter = the distance around the rim of a polygon
Quadrilateral = a polygon with four sides
Parallelogram = a quadrilateral with two pairs of parallel sides
Parallel lines = lines that extend in the same direction staying the same distance apart
Triangle = a polygon with three sides
Square = a polygon with four sides of the same length, with four right angles
Pentagon = a polygon with five sides
Hexagon = a polygon with six sides
Right angle = an angle that has a measurement of 90 degrees
Circle = a plane figure bounded by a single curved line equidistant from every point at the center of the circle
Circumference = the distance around a circle
Diameter = the distance across the center of a circle
Radius = the distance from the center of a circle to any point on the circle
Even numbers = numbers divisible by two (2, 4, 6, 8, 10, etc.)
Odd numbers = numbers not divisible by two (1, 3, 5, 7, 9, etc.)
Decimal = of or based on the number ten (10)
Decimal fraction = a number with one or more numbers to the right of the decimal point
Decimal point = a period between numbers to create a decimal fraction
Million = 1,000,000
Billion = 1,000,000,000
Trillion = 1,000,000,000,000
Quadrillion = 1,000,000,000,000,000
Quintillion = 1,000,000,000,000,000,000
Sextillion = 1,000,000,000,000,000,000,000
Septillion = 1,000,000,000,000,000,000,000,000

Octillion = 1,000,000,000,000,000,000,000,000,000
Horizontal line = a straight line that runs across from left to right, or right to left
Vertical line = a straight line that runs straight up and down, or down and up
Kilometer = a unit of length that equals approximately six-tenths (.6) of a mile
Mile = a unit of length that equals approximately one and six-tenths (1.6) of a kilometer
Cube = a three-dimensional figure with six square faces all the same size

WHAT KINDS OF WORD PROBLEMS CAN YOUR PUPIL EXPLORE?

Type the following story. Ask your pupil to read it to you. Every word she is not able to read should be learned by tracing it. When all the words are known, have her read the story again as many times as she wants and encourage her to tell you how she is working out the solution.

If your pupil wishes, let her add this story to her three-hole notebook. Encourage her to illustrate the story and, if she wishes, show with her illustrations how the problem can be solved.

The Two Farmers

Farmer Bill said to Farmer Sam, "If you will sell me seven acres of your farmland, I will have twice as much land as you."

Farmer Sam said to Farmer Bill, "If you will sell me seven acres of your farmland, I will have just as much land as you."

Who had the most land, Farmer Bill or Farmer Sam?
How much farmland did Farmer Bill have?
How much farmland did Farmer Sam have?

Hmm, should I or shouldn't I give you the answer? Bill, 49 acres; Sam, 35 acres.

Here is another story, a classic. It comes in several varieties, and it would be good for you and your pupil to make up one of your own. Type the story on a sheet of the three-hole notebook paper. Again, as your pupil reads the story for the first time, any word she cannot read easily should be learned by tracing; then, when all words have been traced, do the reading again.

Going across the River

A farmer on his way to market to sell a fox, a goose, and an open basket of corn comes to a river. The small boat he can use to cross the river has room for him and just one of the other three items.

If he takes the corn and leaves the fox with the goose, the fox will eat the goose.

If he takes the fox and leaves the goose and the corn, the goose will eat the corn.

How can he get them all across the river and to the market?

How many trips back and forth across the river will it take?

Surely, I don't need to tell you that one way is for the farmer to take the goose on the first trip, leaving the fox and the corn on the other side. Then, he could take the fox across, and return with the goose, so that the fox wouldn't have the goose to eat. And so on. How about getting a wolf, a goat, and a cabbage across the river?

This is a good story for your pupil to illustrate. Also, it is a base for several good stories using a variety of items to take across the river.

Season with Mathematics throughout the Lessons 53

> **Note:** You won't want to use more than one of these word problems in a single lesson, and you might want to put several days between.

The next story calls for a diagram to show the frog's progress. Three up, two down; repeat, three more up, and two down, and so forth. Warning! Your pupil may figure out the answer quickly, without explaining what she has done. That's just fine. Encourage your pupil to make up a similar problem, and this time write out both the problem and the way to figure the answer. You might reserve a section of the three-hole notebook for similar word problems, complete with illustrated solutions.

The Frog in the Well

A frog has fallen into the bottom of a well 40 feet deep. Every day he jumps up three feet and at night he falls back two feet. How many days will it take the frog to get out of the well?

Six nines make 100. Recall the work you did when you counted to 10 using four 3s and only four 3s. Talk over with your pupil the restrictions in using only the number nine, and encourage her to think about using fractions made up solely of nines. The answer, of course, is: $100 = 99 + (99 \div 99)$.

Here's another story for you to type on three-hole paper in a large font. Again, your pupil reads, traces any new words, and reads again sharing with you how she is figuring out the answer.

> **The Sheep and the Turkeys**
>
> Farmer John has both sheep and turkeys on his farm. His daughter, Mary, counted all the heads and all the feet, and discovered there were 99. She also counted the number of sheep and the number of turkeys and found that there were twice as many turkeys as there were sheep. She took this word problem to school and asked her classmates to tell her how many sheep and how many turkeys were on her farm.

You would, of course, start with the fact that each turkey has one head and two feet, and that each sheep has one head and four feet. Can you take it from there? Remember, there are half as many sheep as turkeys.

You might suggest that your pupil use two kinds of counting items, the one to represent the 5-item sheep and the other to represent the 3-item turkeys until he reaches 99 items. (I suppose you want to know that the answer is nine sheep, and twice as many turkeys!)

> Reach 100 using—only once—each number from zero to nine.

Here's the answer: $50\frac{1}{2} + 49\frac{38}{76} = 100$.

When you use this word problem, your pupil needs to know that it will take fractions to create the answer. Perhaps you should give your pupil the problem of how to make the 10 numerals add up to 100, and make no suggestions, watching what she does and listening to her talking it through. Encourage the discussion.

This is a fun short story, "fun" because the "row" is only three-children long. Primary students who are regularly placed in long lines will especially appreciate this problem.

> **How Many Children in the Row?**
>
> Ann was asked how many children she had lined up. She answered, "Well, there are two children ahead of one child. And there are two children behind one child. And there is one child in the middle."

Did Ann give you enough information so that you can be sure exactly how many children are in the row?

If she did, how many children are there? (three)

You might ask your pupil to use the counting items to represent each child.

This story provides a good way to learn the meaning of such words as "ahead," "behind," "middle," "enough," and "exactly." These words should create a picture for your pupil, and thinking about the row described in the story will help her solve it.

> **Note:** Solving problems like this using counting items is another way to combine kinesthetic, visual, and oral learning methods to reach the answer.

> **Wicked Hard Puzzle**
>
> Take six (only six!) straws or pencils or sticks and arrange them so they form four equal triangles.

Hint: Answer is three-dimensional!

A 50/50 Chance

How many pupils would have to be in a classroom so that there is a 50/50 chance that two of them have the same birthday?

The answer is 23. Your pupil might be allowed to visit some 20 classes in the school to ask if there are any "same-date" birthdays, and figure out whether 10 of the classes had such a pair; that is, whether the answer came to a 50/50 ratio, or whether it was a 9/11 or 11/9 ratio of rooms with same-date birthdays to rooms without.

Which Came First?

[Your pupil's name here] is standing on the bank of a river. A person on the other side shoots a gun that gives off a puff of smoke. The bullet lands in the water.

Will you see the smoke before you hear the gun go off?
Or will you hear the gun and then see the smoke?
Will you see the bullet land in the water before you hear the sound?
Will you see the spot where the bullet landed after or before you heard the sound?

This is a really good story to type and place in the three-hole notebook. It has good scientific information as its base. Did you know that light travels faster than sound, and that sound travels faster than a bullet?

When you write this word problem, use your pupil's name, and perhaps if you know a friend of your pupil, who might shoot a gun, use that person's name. If there is a river or body of water nearby, use that name. In other words, use the story to develop word recognition for family names and familiar locations.

Type this story for your pupil using his name and a particular food, like peanut-butter cookies or apples.

Eating Your Math Lesson

After buying a bunch of [food choice], [pupil's name] ate a third of them on Monday. On Tuesday, [pupil's name] ate half of the remaining [food choice]. On Wednesday, [pupil's name] had only two [food choice] left. How many did [pupil's name] have to begin with?

Herein

What six words can you find in the word "herein," using the letters in the same order as they appear in this word? Starting from the beginning letter "h," "he," of course, is first, and the last word is "in." Can you find the other four?

It would be ideal to use other words and find within them more than one word. The purpose, of course, is to teach your pupil to become a better sight reader, to concentrate on the combinations of letters that form words.

Use the word "herein" in the sandbox, and have your pupil locate the six words, and place each one in the sand: "he"; "her"; "here"; "ere"; "rein"; and "in."

Will take a visit to the dictionary, most probably, for "ere" and "rein."

The month "March" in the sandbox will yield "Ma," and "mar," and "arch."

This is not work for early lessons, and for some kinesthetic learners it may not be useful. Try it; see if your pupil finds the connections. If not, don't use.

This is an old chestnut, but beloved by children. Type the following question in story form, and note how quickly your pupil guesses the answer.

Dirt and a Hole

How much dirt is there in a hole 18 inches square and one foot deep?

I assure you, most pupils will want to do a picture or diagram, and will look forward to asking a younger child to answer that question or one based on his own dimensions. Answer: In the hole, there is no dirt!

Dots and Lines

Draw four dots in two rows one inch apart on the chalkboard.

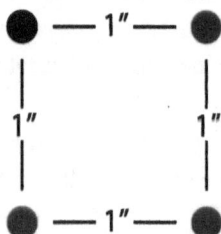

Starting with the left dot in the top row, draw three straight lines, ending up where you started and passing though each dot.

This may take your pupil a few tries, which makes it good to use the chalk. Once done, have your pupil write the puzzle and show the answer in the three-hole notebook.

In this word problem, the goal is to end up with an odd number of baby goats in each pen.

You might use straws to create pens and counting items to stand for the goats.

Now, eventually, your pupil is going to put three goats in each of three pens and then put the fourth pen around all the other pens, and that's how your pupil will end up with an odd number of goats in each of the four pens.

You don't want to give this solution away too quickly. And it may be that your pupil, once having put three "baby goats" in three pens, will figure out what to do with the fourth pen. Again, it's good to use chalk for this so that mistakes can be quickly erased.

It's up to you how much of this story you want to write to frame this word problem. Following is one possible version:

How I Put Nine Baby Goats into Four Pens

Once upon a time, when I was working for Farmer Bill, my job was to put nine baby goats into four pens. Farmer Bill told me I could make the pens any size I wanted, but that he wanted an odd number of baby goats in each pen, and he wanted me to use all four pens. Now, that means I couldn't have two or four or six or eight baby goats in a pen. I could have one or three or five or seven or nine. Here is what I did . . .

> **Two Indians**
>
> Once upon a time, two Indians were walking down the road together. One was a big Indian. One was a little Indian. The little Indian was the son of the big Indian. Yet, the big Indian was not the father of the little Indian.
>   Why?

Does your pupil—as I do—have a German background? Substitute "Germans" for "Indians." Is he Irish, or Mexican? Answer: Of course you know that the two are mother and son, not father and son.

Here's a problem that's particularly good for kinesthetic learners.

> **Number Series**
>
> What is the law behind the following number series? 1, 2, 3, 4, ___, 6, 7.
>   Fill in the blank with the correct number.

This is the easiest example of the number series word problem. You set up a line of numbers, and your pupil must first determine what law is behind the series, and then can fill in the blanks correctly. In this problem, the law is "counting by 1s." Thus 2, 4, ___, 8, 10 would be "counting by 2s." Or, you could state the first law by saying, "Add one to each number." And to the second problem, "Add two to each number."

Again, because it is the kinesthetic method that is most useful for your pupil, have him build a simple number series drawing pictures of items to count.

Start with this one: 3, 7, 4, 8, ___, 9, 6, ___.

First help your pupil establish the law governing the series. What is added to the first number to get the second? Is that the same number added to the third number to get the fourth?

Help your pupil notice that the first and third numbers are just one number apart; so should this be the case with the second and fourth numbers? Are there perhaps two laws in force in this one series? 3, 7, 4, 8, 5, 9, 6, 10.

Use this series problem for your pupil to write a story. Have her set up the series, state the law or laws used to create the series, and then give the answers. Don't just talk out the solution. But after talking it out, have the pupil not only write the solution in words, but also give the correct series in numbers.

If you want your pupil to keep developing number relationships, extend the series for a longer distance, perhaps another 10 numbers.

Here is another simple series: 7, 8, 5, 6, ___, ___.

This is a good series for your pupil to learn how to determine the law behind the series. Should the last two numbers be 3 and 4? Why, or why not?

As soon as you think she can, have your pupil first state a law and then develop a series that follows the law. Have her make up a series leaving some blanks for a relative or friend to work out the answer.

How Old Is Mary?

On Mary's birthday she learned that her mother was four times as old as she was. "Mother," she asked, "will you always be four times as old as I am?"

"Goodness, no," her mother replied. "Why, Mary, in just six years I will only be three times as old as you."

Ben, who was a guest at the birthday party said, "I can figure out how old you are now, Mary, just by what your mother said. You are ___."

To help your pupil figure out what Ben did, use an "x" for Mary's age and "y" for her mother's; hence $4x = y$. Now help your pupil formulate the next algebraic statement since Mary will be $x + 6$, and that $3(x + 6)$ will equal her mother's age shown as $y + 6$.

SEND + MORE = MONEY

Substitute a single digit or number for the letters:
D, E, M, N, O, R, S, Y.

$$\begin{array}{r} SEND \\ + MORE \\ \hline MONEY \end{array}$$

Of course, use one number for "S," another for "E" and so on.

WHAT ARE OTHER WAYS FOR YOUR PUPIL TO LEARN MATH TERMS?

Reading and Writing Geometric Shapes

Teach your pupil how to read and write geometric shapes and terms—for example, the word "triangle." You might first have your pupil draw a simple triangle, then look throughout the room to discover other triangles and explore a math book looking for triangles of various shapes.

After such visual exploration, have your pupil trace the word "triangle" in the sand tray. Perhaps have her draw a simple triangle there at the same time. Teach the word by having your pupil trace over the black crayon word, write it in the air, write it on the chalkboard, and finally put it on an index card. Explore the creating of triangles by dividing squares and rectangles into triangles.

Follow the same steps to learn the word "rectangle." And the word "parallelogram." And the word "circumference." And "diameter." And "circle." Have your pupil illustrate each word on her index cards. Practice, if needed, on scrap paper.

Don't restrict yourself to math terms used in the primary grades. Help your pupil to get ahead of the curve (I apologize for the pun), and teach the terms she will be faced with as she progresses through elementary and junior high math.

If you teach your pupil how to find the distance around a circle, be sure that the "circle" index card contains this information, and perhaps an example.

Similarly, teach your pupil how to find perimeters and areas in each of the different shapes, and include this information on the index cards.

Using graph paper to draw shapes and to estimate and then calculate perimeter or area is especially useful for your kinesthetic learner.

Then, too, show fractions by dividing actual things. There is much to be learned from a simple 8.5 x 11 inch blank sheet of paper cut in half, then each half in half, then each fourth in half, and variations of this.

Your pupil should not only do the cutting (or tearing) of the paper for all math terms, but should always record what she has done. Get her to write full sentences. If it's appropriate, turn some of this work into a story. Ask for illustrations or diagrams.

Graphing

Teach your pupil to graph math-related information. You can get much help from whatever almanac you have for her to use for research. For example, have your pupil

- take a set of statistics and graph it vertically, then perhaps horizontally, or

- do a line graph with a set of statistics, then put the same information into a pie graph.

You can imagine how delighted a kinesthetic learner will be to learn how to take abstract information and through graphing make it demonstrable.

Maps

Another wonderful help for teaching words and exploratory math is a local map. The kinesthetic learner will appreciate that distances between specific locations are marked by a symbol of some kind, along with an actual number standing (in the United States) for miles.

> **Question:** Starting from your house, and going by the way of x, how many miles is it to y?

First, of course, encourage your pupil to trace the route with his finger. Help him locate the symbols indicating distance markers. If needed, use the counting items to add up the distance.

With one pupil, after we had been working with a local map for a couple weeks, I played a kind of How Fast Can You Find It? game. I would say the name of a place and then time (in seconds) how long it took the pupil to point to the exact place. As soon as he got good at finding one location, I then called for finding two on the way to a third.

Soon I was giving him a new map of a nonlocal area. I would give him 10 minutes to locate the names of the towns, then I would time how quickly he could point to them as I called them out. Then I would ask him to locate mountains by name; then to tell me which of those mountains was the highest.

You use the map however you choose. What you are working on is word recognition.

And remember: This isn't a visually learning student, so you want him to locate some places, put his finger on them, say their names, and become familiar not only with their location on the map, but their spelling. Your student needs to build visual learning skills based on his kinesthetic learning skills.

WHAT ARE SOME SAMPLE MATH PROBLEMS USING MAPS AND GRAPHS?

Around the World

First ask your pupil to look at a globe of the world and guess which countries appear to be the largest, next largest, perhaps the top ten. Ask helpful questions. After the estimating, locate the correct answers. Then draw a simple graph, perhaps a horizontal bar graph illustrating the different sizes in square feet or square kilometers.

Other possible questions regarding size of countries:

Which seems larger, Russia or the United States?
Which seems larger, China or Japan?
Which seems larger, Australia or Indonesia? (particularly difficult!)
Does Canada have more land than the United States?

You could do a similar lesson with the longest rivers: the Nile, Amazon, Yangtze, Mississippi-Missouri, and so forth.

The largest lakes are also possible to guess by looking at a globe. The largest lake, the Caspian Sea in Central Asia, is some four and a half times as large as the second largest lake, Lake Superior, which straddles Canada and the United States. This comparison would make a good bar graph; in fact, it would make two good bar graphs—one vertical and one horizontal, each showing the largest eight or nine lakes.

Children often enjoy learning about gold and where it is produced. Following are the top 10 producers: South Africa, United States, Australia, China, Canada, Russia, Peru, Indonesia, Uzbekistan, and Papua New Guinea.

1. Have your pupil locate each nation on a world globe.
2. Have your pupil find in a reference book how many tons of gold were produced in each of the 10 nations in the last three years.
3. Have your pupil graph this information.
4. Have your pupil make up a story (fiction or nonfiction) about the finding, storing, or shipping of gold.

Another "gold" is given at the Olympic games. Again, help your pupil find the answers to the following questions, then use the information by writing a story about it, tracing unknown words.

1. Put these nations in order from the most to the least gold medals in the most recent summer Olympics: Canada, United States, United Kingdom (Britain), Italy, France, Germany, and Russia.
2. Has Sweden or Norway won the most gold medals in the winter Olympics?
3. Has Germany, the United States, or Russia won the most gold medals in the winter Olympics?
4. Has Japan won more than China?

Oil production, particularly as it affects the cost of the gasoline used in the family car, is often a current topic. To include Iraq, you will need to have your pupil find the top fifteen producers.

Large City Population

Of the 30 cities in the world with the largest populations in the year 2005, only 3 were in the United States: New York, Los Angeles, and Chicago. Here are some suggestions for helping your pupil learn about these large cities and their populations:

1. Help your pupil find a source for the populations of the three cities. The Economist *Pocket World in Figures* 2005 edition gives 18.5 million for New York, 12.1 million for Los Angeles, and for Chicago, 8.7 million.
2. A U.S. map and/or a large world globe would be helpful for your pupil to locate each of these cities. Remember to let your pupil put her finger on each city, locating it by hand as well as by eye.
3. You probably don't want to have your pupil trace all the words needed to get a grasp of both the data and the task of creating three graphs. "Population," "New York," "Los Angeles," and "Chicago" are necessary. Perhaps the word "million" as well.
4. You will want to talk about what is meant by "population." And explore a bit just how many a "million" is.

Show your pupil how to present these three cities and their populations in a horizontal bar graph (chart 6.1). Talk it over; for example, you could ask, "Do you want to have the city with the largest be the bottom bar or the top bar?"

Chicago: 8.7 million
Los Angeles: 12.1 million
New York: 18.5 million

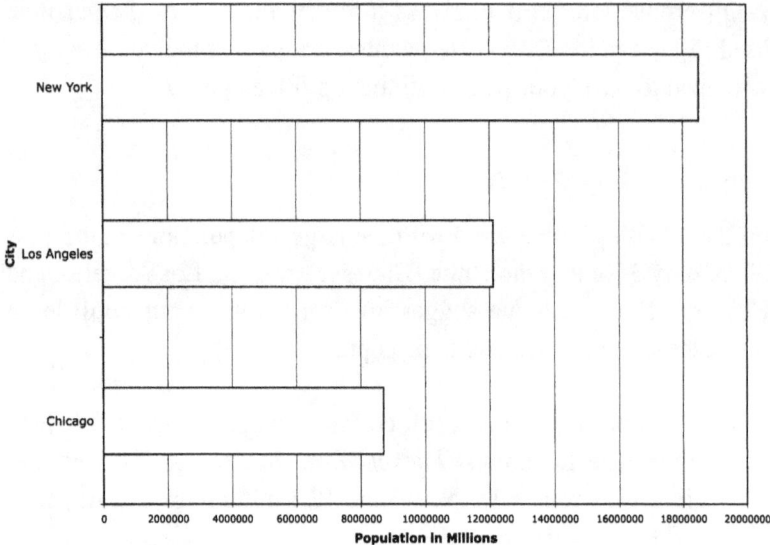

Chart 6.1 Horizontal Bar Graph

Show your pupil how to present these three cities and their populations in a vertical bar graph (chart 6.2):

New York: 18.5 million   Los Angeles: 12.1 million   Chicago: 8.7 million

Show your pupil how to present these three cities and their populations in a line graph, placing the cities in alphabetical order (chart 6.3):

Chicago: 8.7 million
Los Angeles: 12.1 million
New York: 18.5 million

New York in 2005 had the third largest population of any city in the world. Ask your student to guess which city had the largest. (Answer: Tokyo, with 35.3 million.) And ask your pupil to guess

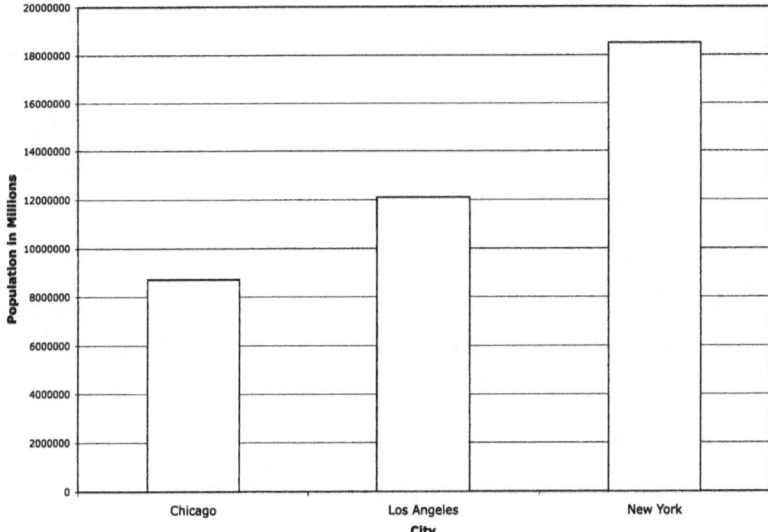

Chart 6.2   Vertical Bar Graph

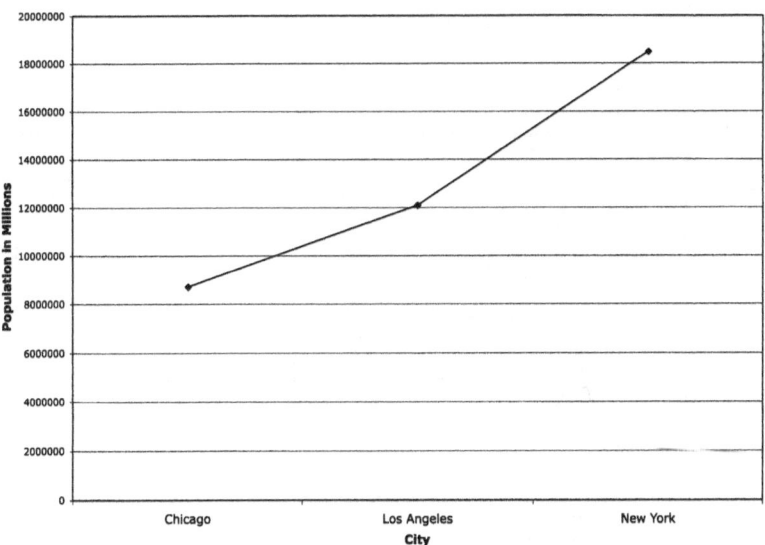

Chart 6.3   Line Graph

which one had the second largest population? (Answer: Mexico City, with 19.0 million.) Locate these three cities on a world map or a globe.

Ask your pupil to make a vertical bar graph showing these three cities, from the one with the smallest population (New York, 18.5 million) to the largest (chart 6.4):

New York: 18.5 million   Mexico City: 19.0 million   Tokyo: 35.3 million

Next, ask your pupil to make a horizontal bar graph showing the three largest cities, from the largest to the smallest (Tokyo, Mexico City, New York; see chart 6.5):

Tokyo: 35.3 million   Mexico City: 19.0 million   New York: 18.5 million

At some other time, you might return to the vertical bar graph for the three largest cities, and add two more: Los Angeles and Chicago.

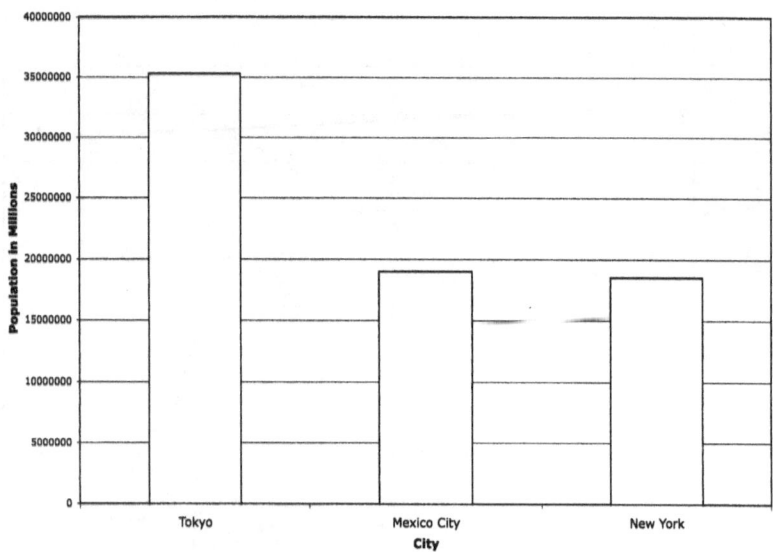

Chart 6.4   Vertical Bar Graph

Season with Mathematics throughout the Lessons 71

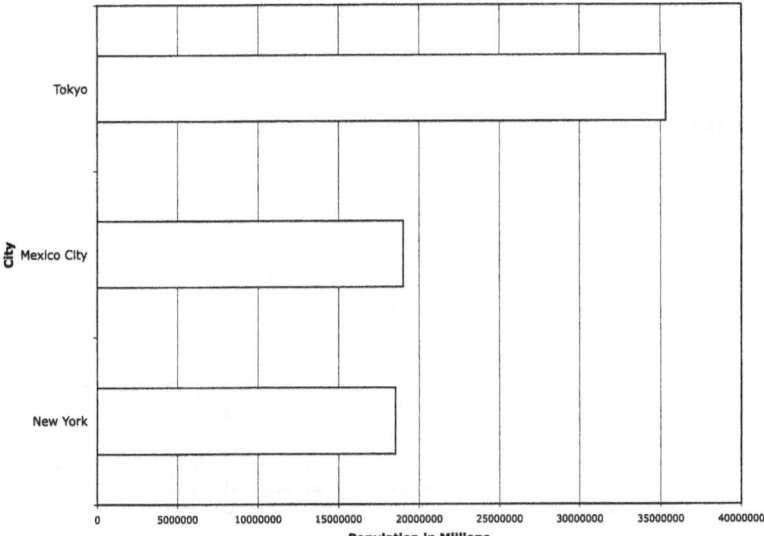

Chart 6.5 Horizontal Bar Graph

If you do so, have your pupil put the five cities in a list with their population figures beside them. Also have your pupil decide how to design the new vertical bar graph. Will your pupil want to use figures of people based on hundreds or thousands or millions? Have your pupil wrestle with the fact that the population is in the millions. Help your pupil see that Tokyo needs to show 35.3 million and Chicago only 8.7 million (see chart 6.6).

Help your pupil figure out how to arrange the graph so that it will show a more than 26-million person population difference. You might help her locate similar graphs and study how they have been commercially done.

Tokyo: 35.3 million   Mexico City: 19.0 million   New York: 18.5 million
        Los Angeles: 12.1 million   Chicago 8.7 million

Once your pupil has learned all about populations and graphs, it would be a special treat for her to go to a first-grade class and, using

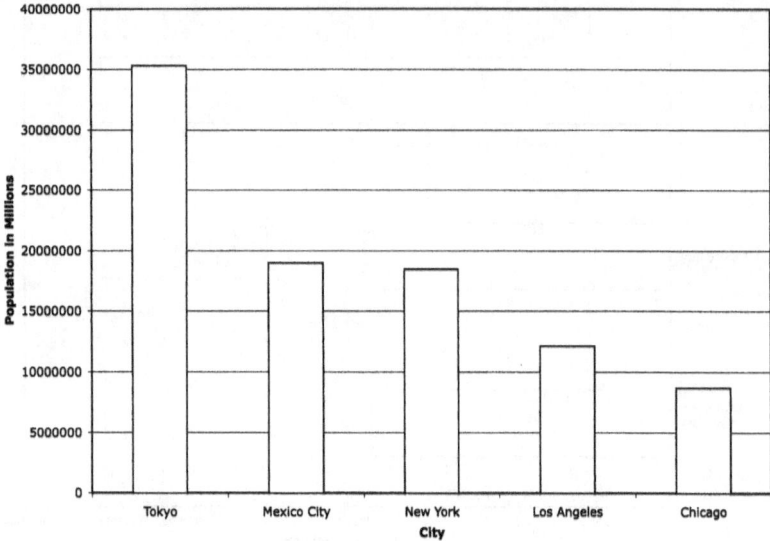

Chart 6.6 Vertical Bar Graph

> **Note:** You would not be researching this information and making these graphs all in one lesson period. Instead, you want to build on your pupil's understanding of graph design in one lesson, expect and encourage more input from the pupil the second lesson, and so on.

the chalkboard, explain about city populations and actually draw one of the graphs complete with the labels. Before your pupil does this "show and tell" lesson, you should make sure that your pupil has command of the necessary words and has practiced making that graph several times.

Lake Sizes

Three of the largest lakes in the world are in the United States. They are, in order of size, Lake Superior, Lake Michigan, and Lake

Huron. Help your pupil locate them on a globe or large United States map, and note that two of them share space in both Canada and the United States. Of course, encourage your pupil to put her finger directly on the lakes, making sure to find the name of each lake.

A map of the state of Michigan may be best to show the dividing line between Canada and the United States.

Help your pupil discover how large each one is in square miles in a reference book. Use the data for each whole lake, explaining that some of the water space is in Canada, and some in the United States. Rounded off the sizes are as follows:

Lake Superior: 81,000 square miles
Lake Huron: 77,900 square miles
Lake Michigan: 74,700 square miles

Again, you will want your pupil to use the sand tray to trace the word "lake." Also "Superior," "Huron," and "Michigan." It's up to you whether you want to use the abbreviation for "square," but you will want to have your pupil trace "sq." or "square," and "mile."

Before helping your pupil trace a finger around each of the lakes, point out how most of the roads near the water are not wide interstate highways, but smaller roads, often a black line on the map and not a red line. Help your pupil understand the legend for the map you are using, then get the pupil to make the connection between what is shown in the legend and what appears on the map.

Sometimes it is very helpful for your pupil to put one finger on a symbol in the legend, and a finger from the other hand on its location on the map itself.

Note: For the kinesthetic learner to understand relative size, it would be very helpful for her to use tracing paper and a dark pencil, trace the outlines for the three lakes, and notice by putting one over another the differential in size. It dramatizes the size of Superior and clarifies the closeness in size of Lake Huron and Lake Michigan.

You may want to help your pupil cut out the outline on the tracing paper of each lake. Then transfer that outline to a stiffer piece of paper. This will allow you to help your pupil place the name on each outlined lake. It also will make it possible to use the lake drawings more than once.

Now, help your pupil draw a horizontal bar graph so that it looks like water in the bars, and let your pupil decide which lake should appear at the bottom of the graph, which in the middle, and which on top.

The graph included here does not show "water," and has the largest as the top bar (chart 6.7).

Lake Superior: 81,000 square miles
Lake Michigan: 74,700 square miles
Lake Huron: 77,900 square miles

Is Lake Superior larger than your state? Interesting question. It is the kind of question most children like. Some companion questions:

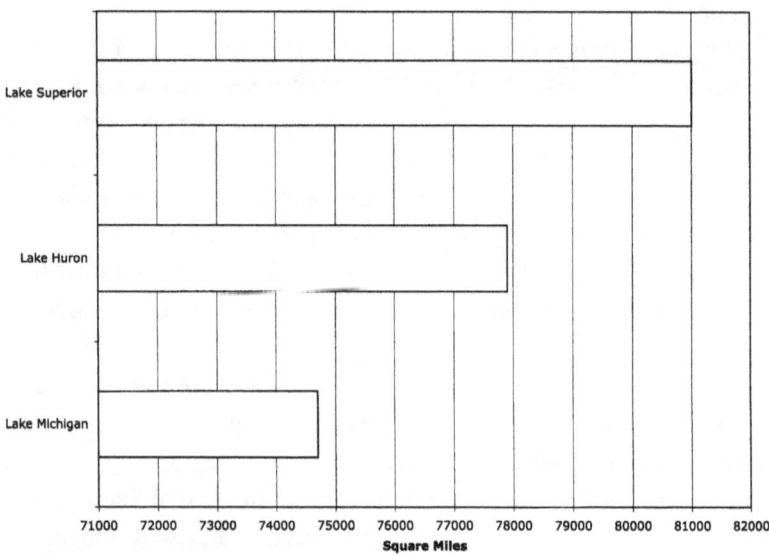

Chart 6.7 **Horizontal Bar Graph**

> **Note:** This is also a good time to teach your pupil what a "square mile" is. Perhaps you will want to have her draw a four-inch line with a ruler, then at a 90-degree angle draw another four-inch line, and repeat that until the pupil has created a 4-inch open square. Help her draw other-color or faint lines dividing the four-inch square into four one-inch squares. This may help your pupil understand what it means that Lake Superior's watery surface covers 81,000 square miles.

- How many states have more square miles of land and water than Lake Superior? (And it is "superior" for tutors of the kinesthetic way because their pupils want to learn how to read the names of the states to discover the answer.)
- Which states have more square miles of land and water than Lake Superior's all-water area? Of course, Texas is one of them.

An excellent project is to make a tracing of the outer edges of Lake Superior, and make a similar tracing of the outer boundaries of your state from the same map. Then place the tracing of Lake Superior over the tracing of your state to determine which one is larger and which one is smaller in area.

Why from the same map? Because the distances are equivalent.

Even if your state is California, which has a different shape than the lake, which one is larger is still fairly obvious. What about New York State?

Statistics for Your Own State

You want to get a good road map for your state.

I shall use Vermont as one example. I lived there for 37 years in a one-room schoolhouse built in 1874 and tutored many of the local children in the kinesthetic way.

And I will use Arizona, as that's where I have lived since September 10, 2001. It's also where I wrote this book.

Interstate Highways

Arizona has how many federal interstate highways?
Which one covers the shortest distance in Arizona?
Which one covers the longest distance in Arizona?

You might ask similar questions as your pupil studies a map of the state in which she lives. I am using Arizona (and Vermont) only as an "example," so that you will have some suggestions for ways to use a highway map to enhance your pupil's reading and math skills. The answers for Arizona follow:

Interstate 15, about 40 miles
Interstate 19, about 60 miles
Interstate 17, about 140 miles
Interstate 8, about 180 miles
Interstate 40, about 360 miles
Interstate 10, about 380 miles

Your pupil should locate each of the interstate number symbols for her state. She should trace with a finger along each full route before looking for the numbers designating miles between the mile markers. Let your pupil get familiar with how to follow an interstate route, and since you are working with a map for your own state, help your pupil identify the major towns and cities through which each interstate highway passes. Expect your pupil to want to do the tracing several times. Have her talk about what is being traced while she is doing the tracing; for example, "I am starting in Flagstaff, Arizona, and I am going to go south on I 10 to Tucson."

Help your pupil make a horizontal bar graph projecting the length of all of your state's interstate highways. Here's a graph for the six

> **Note:** Is it true that if an interstate highway has an even number (like 8, 40, and 10) that it mainly goes east/west? Is it true that interstate highways with an odd number (like 15, 19, and 17) generally go north/south?

interstate highways in Arizona (chart 6.8). You might have your pupil check these statistics. Maybe I (Interstate) 10 is not longer than I 40 across Arizona.

I 15: 40 miles
I 19: 60 miles
I 17: 140 miles
I 8: 180 miles
I 40: 360 miles
I 10: 380 miles

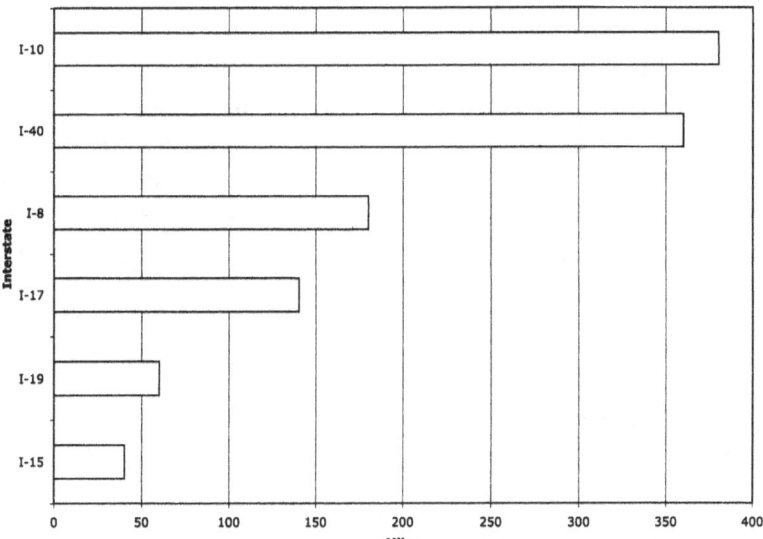

Chart 6.8 Horizontal Bar Graph

Summit and Mountain Heights

Explain that the word "summit" on a road map usually means a high point on a highway, not the height of a mountain named "summit."

Show your pupil the "legend" for the map you are using and help her find the symbol for a mountain—most often, a small triangle peak at the top. For this activity, we will stay on the far eastern side of my state (Arizona), but for your state, presuming there are some mountains, choose an area where there are several.

Use the sand tray perhaps to show that "ft." is the abbreviation for "feet." It is good for your pupil to create in the sand tray both the full word (feet) and the abbreviation (ft.) if there is room. It's possible that the map you are using does not use lowercase "feet," but uppercase "FEET." If so, use the sand tray to teach "FEET" and the abbreviation "FT."

Mountain peaks in a state like Arizona are fun for the pupil to locate, since Arizona is known for its desert land, not mountains, and for having the deepest canyon in the United States. If your pupil is not interested in Arizona, then there is no reason to study its mountains; move on to your own state.

First, help your pupil find the symbol for a mountain peak in the legend, then begin making a list of the mountain peaks on the eastern border of Arizona from north to south, listing each one's elevation. Next, after your pupil has found several or all of the peaks, help her reorder them by height—lowest to highest, or vice versa—and then create a vertical bar graph, perhaps using thin "peak" triangles instead of rectangular bars. My list of Arizona peaks follows.

Pastora Peak: 9,412 feet
Escudilla Mountain: 10,912 feet
Rose Peak: 8,786 feet
Maple Peak: 8,294 feet
Mitchell Peak: 7,951 feet
Maverick Mountain: 6,901 feet

Flys Peak: 9,666 feet
Chiricahua Peak: 9,759 feet
Swisshelm Mountain: 7,185 feet

Please note that these nine mountains are not listed in either alphabetical order or in order of height. Purpose: Have your pupil create such specialized lists. Here is one such list based on the heights in feet of the nine mountains.

Maverick Mountain: 6,901 feet
Swisshelm Mountain: 7,185 feet
Mitchell Peak: 7,951 feet
Maple Peak: 8,294 feet
Rose Peak: 8,786 feet
Pastora Peak: 9,412 feet
Flys Peak: 9,666 feet
Chiricahua Peak: 9,759 feet
Escudilla Mountain: 10,912 feet

Using this student-generated list, have your pupil create a horizontal bar graph; then, a vertical bar graph. Discuss which graph seems to create a clearer picture of the sizes of the mountains. Determine together whether to start the height numbers at 6,000 feet, and end the graph at 11,000 feet. Certainly you would not want to start at a height of one foot!

Next, using a map of the state in which your pupil lives, have her select a group of mountains (if there are any), and after making a list, develop a similar horizontal bar graph.

Here are some questions for your student to answer about Arizona's mountains:

1. Is Escudilla Mountain (10,912 ft.) the highest in the state?
2. If it isn't, what mountain is the highest? (Answer: Humphreys Peak [12,633]).

> **Note:** The handwork to make the graph gives your pupil a better "feel" for learning how to spell, write, and pronounce the necessary words. Perhaps later, when your pupil is fairly through with the need to trace words in the sand tray, you can introduce using the computer's graphic capabilities to help develop better visual learning methods.

To help your pupil find the answers, you might

1. give your pupil the coordinates to find Humphreys Peak (L 9 on the road map I am using; you may need to show your pupil how to use those coordinates to locate sites and to inform others where sites can be found); or
2. give your pupil time to look in sections of the map that are greenish in color indicating wooded areas to locate other mountain peaks and note their heights.

The following information about Vermont's mountains is given as another example of how you might have your pupil research mountains in her own state.

Vermont is known for its Green Mountains. Haystack Mountain, elevation 3,345 feet, is the mountain nearest the southern border of Vermont, and Jay Peak, elevation 3,861 feet, is the most northern. Further east and nearly at the same latitude, are three other mountains: Gore, Sable, and Monadnock.

A good lesson in word recognition is the connecting of symbols used on maps with the actual word for which they are substitutes. Be sure you remember to tell the pupil to look for the small dark triangle as a location marker for a mountain peak. You should also

Season with Mathematics throughout the Lessons 81

warn your pupil that there is a Monadnock Mountain in southern New Hampshire, as well as in Vermont; make sure your pupil locates the correct one.

Now have your pupil locate Gore, Sable, and Vermont's Monadnock mountains, noting their elevations.

Have the pupil make a list of all five, first, alphabetical.

Gore: 3,330 feet
Haystack: 3,345 feet
Jay Peak: 3,861 feet
Monadnock: 3,140 feet
Sable: 2,725 feet

Create a line graph from this information (chart 6.9).

Again, have your pupil make another list by elevation from lowest to highest. Create a line graph from this information. Because the

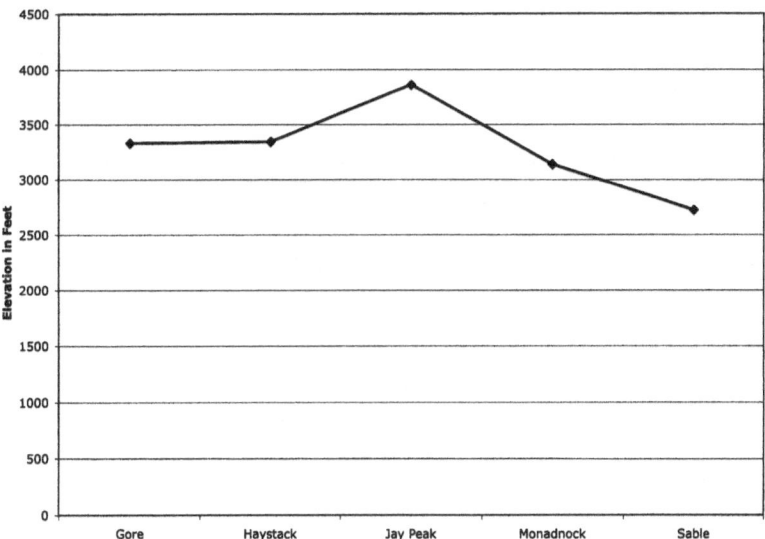

Chart 6.9 Line Graph

lowest height is 2,275 feet and the highest is only 3,861 (less than 1,600 feet difference), a line graph works fairly well (chart 6.10).

Sable: 2,725 feet
Monadnock: 3,140 feet
Gore: 3,330 feet
Haystack: 3,345 feet
Jay Peak: 3,861 feet

Once your pupil has dealt with a small number of locations, as in these mountain peaks, it would be useful to solidify her understanding and reading, writing, computing skills by asking your pupil to locate two more mountain peaks in Vermont. Have your pupil put them in alphabetical order with the known five, provide their heights, and make a vertical bar graph illustrating this information. For example, your pupil could use Camel's Hump, elevation 4,086 feet, and Mount Mansfield, elevation 4,393 feet.

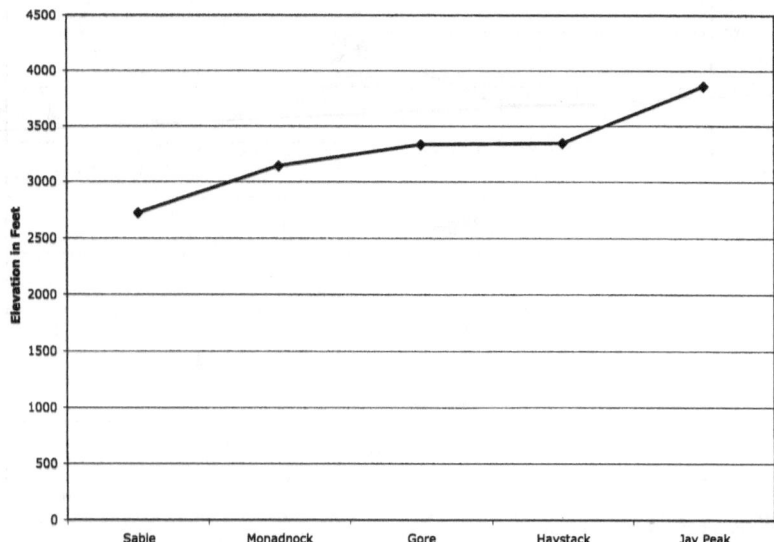

Chart 6.10   Line Graph

State Population

Interestingly, Vermont and Wyoming have the smallest populations of the 50 states. Wyoming has a lot more land, but fewer men, women, and children than Vermont. Help your pupil find the most current population count for these two states.

Let your pupil choose two more states (preferably her own state being one of the two) and make vertical and horizontal bar graphs comparing both square miles of land (one set of graphs; see charts 6.11 and 6.12) and population (another set of graphs; see charts 6.13 and 6.14) for the four states. Here are the graphs with data from an almanac. Population figures are for 2005. I have arbitrarily added Rhode Island and New Hampshire.

Vermont: 9,614 square miles; 621,000 people
Wyoming: 97,814 square miles; 507,000 people
Rhode Island: 1,545 square miles; 1.08 million people
New Hampshire: 9,350 square miles; 1.3 million people

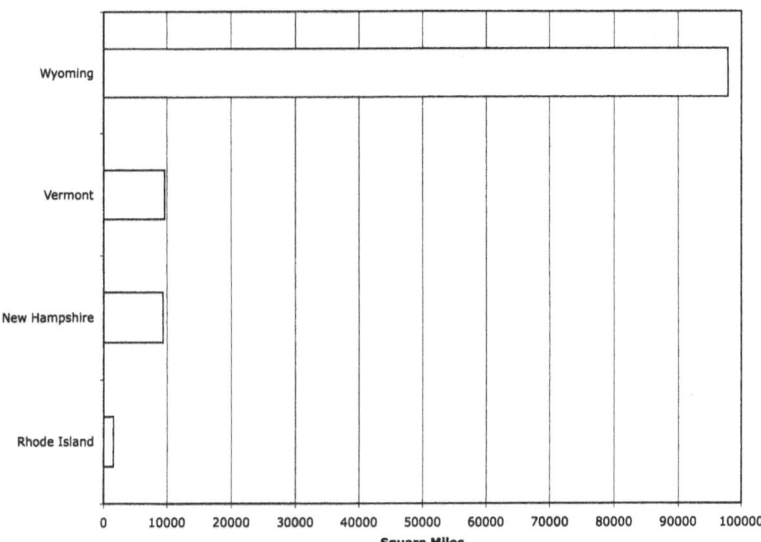

Chart 6.11   Horizontal Bar Graph

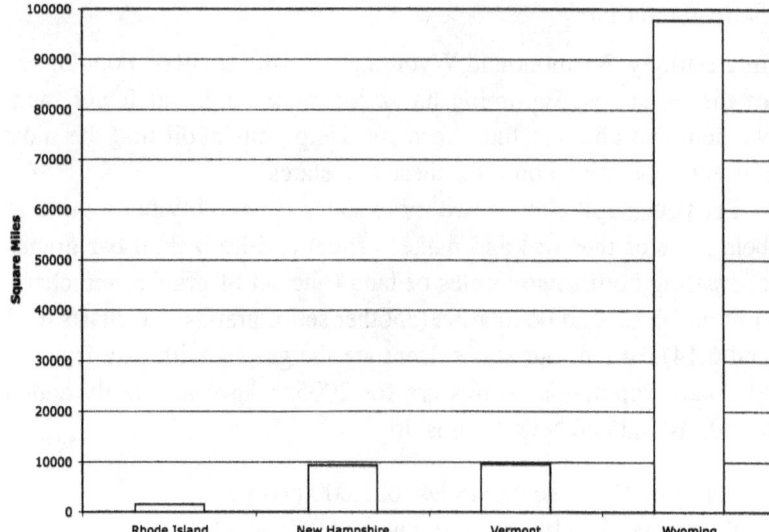

Chart 6.12 Vertical Bar Graph

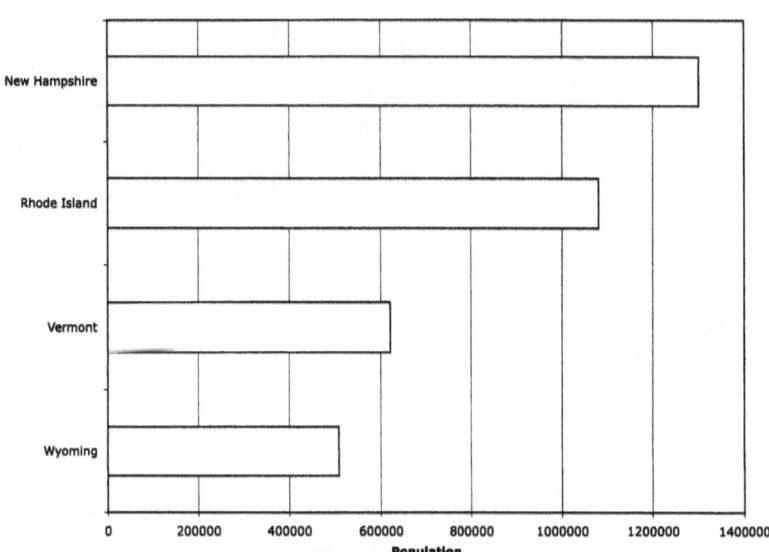

Chart 6.13 Horizontal Bar Graph

Season with Mathematics throughout the Lessons 85

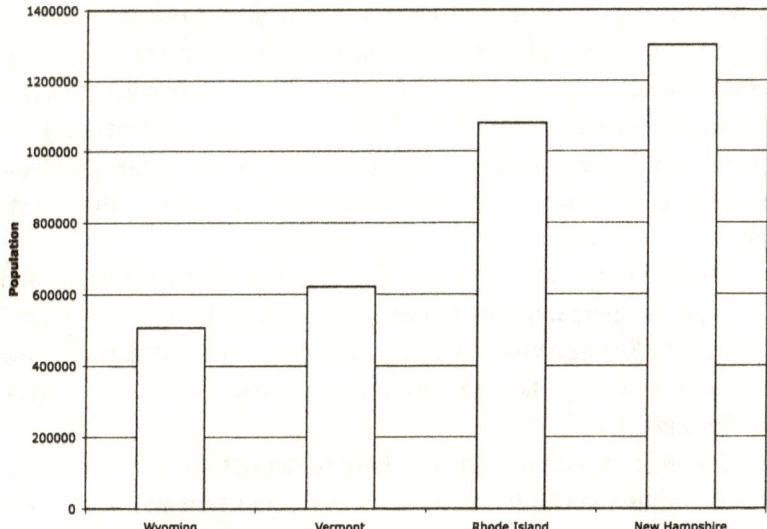

Chart 6.14   Vertical Bar Graph

Here are the graphs, first for square miles, then for population:

Rhode Island: 1,545 square miles
New Hampshire: 9,350 square miles
Vermont: 9,614 square miles
Wyoming: 97,814 square miles
NH: 1.3 million
RI: 1.08 million
VT: 621,000
WY: 507,000

Learning How to Use a Road Map

In Arizona, of course, the Colorado River is the big story, especially the forming of the Grand Canyon. Unfortunately, the flat map does not do justice to this magnificent world-class wonder, the Grand Canyon, so let's look at the Little Colorado River instead.

If your pupil lives in Arizona, you might start a lesson by asking her to find a very small town named Cameron. Instead of giving coordinates, you might tell her that Cameron is near where Federal Route 89 meets State Route 64. Then explain that in Cameron, your pupil will find a thin blue line depicting the Little Colorado River that has been formed from the melting snow and rain in the mountains to the north.

You might then start a story: "Pretend that you have a canoe and a fellow paddler, and want to head downstream from Cameron until you get to Springerville." Pause in the story, and spend some time showing your pupil how to trace the map's blue line from Cameron to Springerville.

Continue the story: "You will have to get out often and carry the canoe around such obstructions as dams and falls and places too shallow for the canoe. But follow that faint blue line marking the Little Colorado River, and make a note of what towns you go through or pass by very closely. Can you find Sunrise? And further south, Holbrook? What river joins the Little Colorado near the town of Holbrook coming in from the east?"

Point out that the water in Puerco River joins the water in the Little Colorado, making it a larger river as it heads further south. Ask the pupil to find Lyman Dam and Lyman Lake on the south side of the dam.

If you and your pupil really live in Arizona (or have reason to visit there), it would be grand to take a road trip to see (and perhaps even cross on a bridge) the Little Colorado River.

And, of course, a trip to the Grand Canyon might well start at Cameron, where Route 89 meets Route 64. Help your pupil locate Route 64 where it meets I 40 and then trace it north, using her finger, to where it meets Route 89.

Go west on Route 64 and be sure to stop at the several locations along the rim of the Grand Canyon where you are able to see far enough over the edge to get a glimpse of the Colorado River.

Once your pupil has learned to follow a river, suggest routes from one destination to another and ask for a set of roads that would be the shortest route. Ask for a set of roads that would take you over a summit. Ask for a set of roads that will pass near a mountain.

By using your own state map, many of the names will be familiar to your pupil, hence there will be an interest in learning how to read them, spell them, and locate them.

Drawing Driving Maps

The oral/aural learner likes to talk her way through a set of directions to go from one place to another. For example, looking at the Vermont map and describing how to drive north from Chester to Rutland, the oral learner would say (usually aloud), "Go north on Route 103 through Gassets and Ludlow; do not take Route 155 south or Route 140 west, but stay on Route 103, and a few miles south of Rutland, join Route 7 north, which is a four-lane highway, and bear right into the center of town."

The kinesthetic learner would trace that route with a finger, probably saying, either silently to herself or aloud, just what the oral/aural learner says. The kinesthetic learner would note, by pausing, where roads go off from Route 103 (both on the left and the right), feeling the need with her finger to stay on Route 103 until it actually meets Route 7. Then she would trace the turn north (to the right) to the circle and name denoting arrival in Rutland.

A drawing would look like the following map, indicating towns and roads right and left (figure 6.3).

Now help your pupil start in Chester and go to Burlington, the largest city in Vermont. First, of course, help your pupil locate the small town of Chester (where routes 11 and 103 meet), and the city of Burlington over 100 miles northwest of Chester. Be sure you help your pupil discover that Burlington is located on Lake Champlain.

It might be good to ask your pupil to find the routes between Chester and Burlington that use the most interstate highway miles. Again, help your pupil locate the only two interstate highways in

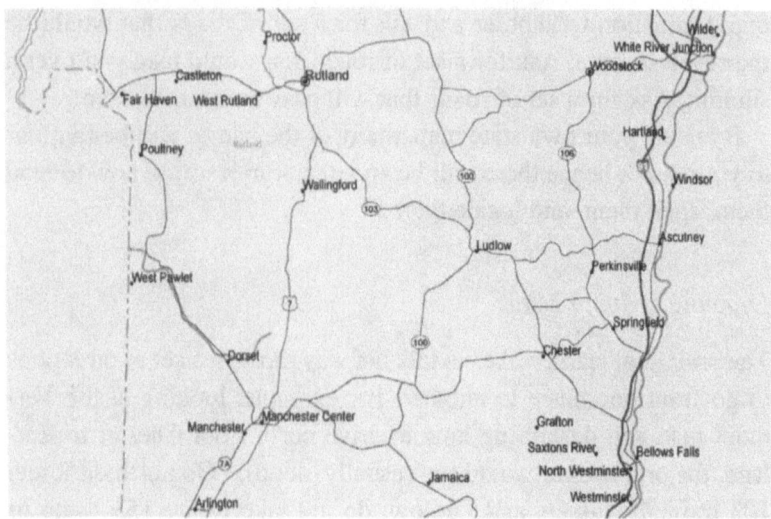

Figure 6.3   Map of Vermont

Vermont, and then help your pupil determine the quickest way to get from Chester on paved roads to first I 91, then onto I 89.

Before having your pupil start describing the route orally, have her trace with a finger, correcting the route as needed, then retrace once more, determining the "best" route. Your pupil might trace a third time, asking herself about the route changes and taking note of busy intersections. Be sure that after "silent" tracing, your pupil says orally what the route is like.

Here's a route from Chester to Burlington:

Take Route 103 north to Route 131 east (right turn).
Take Route 131 east to I 91.
Go north on I 91 (left turn from Route 131), until you reach I 89. That interstate highway passes across I 91.
Go northwest on I 89 (not southeast to New Hampshire), and stay on I 89 until it meets Route 7 in Burlington.

Season with Mathematics throughout the Lessons

Ask your pupil for a drawing—a personal map—for the use of the driver for this one-way trip. But before doing the drawing, be sure to have your pupil come back down south from Burlington to Chester using exactly the same roads you chose for the trip up north to Burlington. In fact, help your pupil go up and down with a finger tracing the route several times. Talk about where the finger is on the route and what the scenery might be like.

You will want to be sure to use the sand tray for the words "north," "south," "east," and "west"; possibly, too, for "Chester" and "Burlington."

When making the drawing, you want to be sure you show your pupil where the routes curve in more than one direction (if they do), and try to show approximate distances. For example, the distance north on I 91 is much shorter than the distance on I 89, and your pupil's map should reflect that difference. The kinesthetic learner should remind herself of that fact when tracing her finger along the route.

> **Note:** There are computer programs that spell out directions. Again, having your pupil use them before she is reading at grade level won't be much help to the kinesthetic learner. But, once a pupil has become fairly proficient at reading a road map and creating pictured and labeled directions, it might be a good time to teach your pupil to use a map program for comparison and to help the pupil recognize how well she can read and compute.

For a different route back to Chester from Burlington, ask your pupil to describe a route that does not include an interstate highway. For example, make sure her finger is on Route 7 in Burlington. Have her slowly move a finger on the other hand south toward Rutland. (One hand might be on the route, the other on Rutland, showing the way south along Route 7.)

What to do in Rutland? First, with one finger on Rutland, locate Chester, and put another finger on that small town. Now talk about all the good choices. Either ask your pupil which direction she wants to take, or ask for the turn east on Route 7 in the center of Rutland. This time, make Woodstock the next destination.

Again, it would be good for your pupil to have the finger on one hand marking Woodstock and a finger on the other hand moving along Route 4 going east. If it were my student, I would ask, "Will any of Route 4 be along a river? Only a Vermonter living in the area would want to learn to pronounce and spell the name of that river!"

But what to do in Woodstock? Have your pupil locate Chester in relation to Woodstock: one finger of one hand on Woodstock; one finger of the other hand on Chester. Of course, this will reveal that you have to go south to Chester. Have your pupil trace each way. Perhaps she could find the set of routes that are the shortest distance in miles, or perhaps you could decide you want to go past Mt. Ascutney or along the Black River.

Have your pupil trace the routes; talk them out; draw them freehand; label rivers, mountains, side roads, cross roads, and any towns through which you will pass.

Ask questions about your pupil's choices. Ask for estimates from your pupil about which set of routes might be shortest in miles, but take more time than another possible set of routes.

Go back up to Burlington: What routes should your pupil trace if you want to go through Rutland?

What routes should your pupil trace if you don't want to go through Rutland?

Now for an example of a difficult question: What routes could you take if you want to go by ferry from Burlington to New York State to reach State Route 373 at Port Kent? What routes south can you take in New York State to get to the ferry at Essex, New York, and cross back over to Vermont to the town of Charlotte? (Vermonters say this word by putting emphasis on the second syllable; that is on "lotte.")

And to continue this more difficult route, ask your pupil to find the route south of Charlotte that will go over Middlebury Gap (road elevation 2,144 feet), and meet Route 100. Again, trace the route on Route 100 south to the town of Ludlow, and from there get back to Chester on Route 103.

You would, of course, be finding progressively complex routes between destinations on the road map most familiar to your pupil.

Here is one more set of suggestions for using any road map to help your pupil to become a successful reader. I am using Vermont only as an example.

You might ask your pupil to look carefully at all the routes between the small town of Chester and the large city of Burlington, noting the many connecting roads going east/west crossing or touching the many north/south roads.

You might specify requirements that would cause your pupil to make a lot of route and direction changes. For example:

- Part of the route must go beside a lake.
- Part of the route must go near a mountain at least 3,000 feet high.
- Part of the route must go where the water in Lake Champlain can be seen.
- Part of the route must be on a road marked "scenic."

Perhaps you will need to have your pupil start with a finger on a possible good route, and then talk about what might be seen from that road. You could talk out a route, noting how your pupil is finding what you are saying by tracing the route correctly.

Again, it is very good to ask the student to trace a chosen route using tracing paper, then transfer to regular paper, with your pupil placing route numbers, intersections, towns, lakes, river, mountains, etc., on the paper.

Special Maps: Subway, Train, Metropolitan Areas

When I was living in Brookline (a suburb of Boston), I was tutoring an eight-year-old who was a strong kinesthetic learner. I had to go by subway (called the "T" by Bostonians) once a week to the Boston Museum of Science where I was taking an evening class. I hired a senior in high school to come each week and meet me and my pupil at a subway entrance on Beacon Street in Brookline. At this stop, the train was above ground.

The pupil was in charge of buying the tickets (asking me for the money for purchase), for choosing the route, and for letting me know where I was to exit in order to go to the Museum. While I was taking the class, my pupil and his substitute tutor were studying the subway map and were taking the trips the pupil was choosing routes to explore.

At our next tutoring session, the pupil traced on the map for me the routes they had taken and drew a rough map of those routes on a city map with his finger—easy when the train was above ground; not so easy when it was underground.

Experiencing the actual routes riding on the train, coupled with the study of both the subway map and the metropolitan city map, helped that pupil gain expertise in both the reading and the math involved in distance and time estimates. At the close of one tutoring session he asked how the subway trains got turned around, or if some cars only went one way and some another. The subway stop nearest where he lived was at street level, with one set of tracks going west and the other set going east, with one-way streets for automobile traffic on either side.

We arranged for him to go with his high school friend to the "end of the line" and learn what happened to the train cars. He couldn't wait to write a story about it, illustrate the story, and share with some younger children.

He became interested in knowing how to read and spell the names of the stations, and more than 40 years later asked me when we spoke by phone at a holiday time, "Is Alewife still a subway stop on the MTA [Boston subway system]?" He loved that combination when he was eight years old: "ale" and "wife," especially when he learned that it wasn't an "ailing" wife!

Metropolitan Maps

These are particularly useful for the pupil who lives in a large metropolitan city or one of its suburbs. The pupil loves finding known places, loves tracing the routes between where she lives and important buildings or intersections of stops for buses or the subway. Exactness is important; hence, there is an incentive to learn to spell place names and specified intersections and names of subway stops correctly. Street names, too, are important for the pupil, and again provide an incentive to make the drawing of a simple map correct and clear.

The child who lives in an apartment building needs to learn how to draw maps to show how to get from that building to a bus route or subway stop; how to get from that building to the school she attends, to the church, to the grocery store, to places to play, to homes of relatives or special friends.

Unique Maps

A zoo. A historic site. The Grand Canyon. A museum. Most of these locations have excellent maps, and wise use of them by a tutor can teach good word recognition and a lot of practical math.

My pupil, who loved the subway research in greater Boston, also loved making a map of the local zoo. It included only the animals he particularly wanted to visit!

HOW CAN YOU USE AN ALMANAC AS A TEACHING TOOL?

In short, an almanac is

- an excellent resource book to teach use of an index,
- an excellent resource book to teach use of a table of contents,
- an excellent source of data to use to create graphs and tables,
- an excellent resource book for information about agencies in the federal government, and
- a good resource for sports information.

Sports

If the pupil you are tutoring lives in Wisconsin, Michigan, California, Florida, Pennsylvania, Oregon, Nebraska, Texas, Illinois, or Ohio, you might have her find the results of the Rose Bowl NCAA football games from 1995–2005, and then ask a series of questions to stimulate accurate reading and a little math:

- Which college football team won more than twice in those ten years? Answer: None. Good question to support careful reading.
- In which year was the score the closest, and which two teams played? Answer: 2005. Texas 38, Michigan 37.
- In which year was the score the widest, and which teams played? Answer: 2002. Miami of Florida 37, Nebraska 14.
- The University of Wisconsin played twice in the Rose Bowl between 1995 and 2005. Did they win both times?

If your pupil lives in a town with a high school football team, teach her how to make a table for 10 years of "final" games somewhat like the table in the almanac or other resource book you are using.

Basketball may be an even more favorite interest for your pupil. Generally an almanac will give the scores for the champions of the NCAA Division 1 men's basketball final four scores. Again, ask questions calling for name recognition and some simple math:

- Between 1995 and 2005, did any team win by just one point?
- Between 1995 and 2005, did any team win by more than 10 points?

And for the student's favorite high school, make a table of all the varsity games, showing opponents and scores.

Does your pupil live in Tennessee, Indiana, Connecticut, or Maryland? Have her find the table for NCAA Division 1 women's basketball championship results. Just look at the results from 1995–2006.

- Which college won the most championships?
- Which one the second most?
- Was the University of Connecticut ever a runner-up during those years?
- Was the University of Tennessee ever a runner-up during those years?
- Which two teams had the closest final score? What year was that?

Cell Phone Growth

In 1990, less than 6 million cell phones were in use in the United States. How many were in use by the year 2000? How many by the year 2005? Have your pupil do some subtraction and perhaps make a table showing just the years from 2001 to 2005. This is the kind of data children love to spring on parents and other friendly adults!

> **Note:** Yes, all this information can be found on the Internet. But it is clearly best for the kinesthetic learner to be able to put her finger directly on the data. It is certainly possible for you to show your pupil, once reading comes fairly easily for her, how to find sports records (and other facts of interest) using the Internet.

Oceans

There are just five of them according to a world agency dealing with water locations. It would be good for your pupil make a table based on the area of each, from the smallest to the largest. It will start with the Atlantic Ocean and end with the Pacific Ocean. Your pupil will find it interesting that the Pacific Ocean's liquid area is greater than all the land area on Planet Earth.

Farms

Perhaps your pupil lives on a farm or in a farm community. Use an almanac chart giving data about the number of farms in 1980, 1990, 2000, and 2004 (or whatever set of four years is in the almanac or resource book you are using). Let your pupil choose 10 of the 50 states and make a table that is not alphabetical, but shows either from the highest or the lowest the changing number of farms over those four years. From the almanac I am using, California had 81,000 in 1980; more farms in 1990 and 2000; and then only 76,000 in 2004. New York started with 47,000 farms in 1980 and lost some each decade, ending up with 36,000 in 2004.

Children's Living Arrangements

You may or may not wish to explore these statistics. Many of our nation's 73-plus million children now live outside the traditional mother, father, and siblings arrangement—sometimes called "married couples with their own children." In 1960, more than 45 percent of all children in the United States lived in two-parent families. Today, less than 25 percent of U.S. children live in two-parent families. Of those who do not, the majority live with a single parent, most with their mother. The statistics for children under age 18 in 2002 show that some 3.7 million of them lived with grandparents.

Race or Hispanic Origin

Certainly if your pupil is a nonwhite, statistics about such ethnicity by states and cities are interesting. An almanac probably won't have the statistics for the area in which your pupil lives unless it is one of the largest metropolitan areas. This will give you an opportunity to help your pupil use research facilities at a local library and learn how to get information by phone from an appropriate government authority.

If your pupil is of Hispanic or Latino origin, perhaps have her make a table of the 10 states with the largest percent of population that is of Hispanic/Latino origin. New Mexico would be at the top (in the year 2002, Hispanics and Latinos were nearly 43 percent of the total population for the state, about 1.9 million). Help your pupil find the next nine, making sure she notes the name or abbreviation for each state and the percent before designing a table or chart.

There is a very important difference between a metropolitan area with a large Hispanic/Latino population in number of persons and a metropolitan area with a large Hispanic/Latino population as a percent of the total population of the area.

For example, in the greater Los Angeles area (population 6.6 million in the year 2000), Hispanic/Latinos were 40.3 percent of the population. This means that there were some 2.7 million Hispanic/Latino people living in that area.

But the city of Laredo, Texas, which had about 182,000 population in 2002, had some 90.3 percent of that population listed as Hispanic/Latino. That is more than twice the percentage for the greater Los Angeles area. Help your pupil note the huge difference in size (population) of Los Angeles from Laredo.

If your pupil is Asian, Black, or Native American, exploring tables with these statistics based on the city in which your pupil lives is generally of great interest. Of course, it is helpful for your pupil to be able to read and write the words attached to her ethnicity. Of special interest, of course, are the divisions of ethnicity in her school, neighborhood, and county.

One of my pupils, after discovering that only a small percent of the population in Hawaii was registered as "Native Hawaiian" and that what he called "a whopping percent" were registered as "Asian," decided to do a lot of research on this 50th state, and most of his information came from his reading and research.

He did his first personal interview when he located someone in his town that had lived in Hawaii. He discovered the old copies of *National Geographic* magazine in his local library and vigorously worked to learn to read them.

He made graph after graph, starting by comparing the size of Hawaii's volcano with several others in the world.

Did we have to build a toy volcano, and make it smoke? Yes.

The Caldecott Medal

This is the prize awarded by the American Library Association (ALA) yearly to the illustrator of a children's book. Many of the books are still in print even though first published years ago.

Fun activity: Choose one Caldecott Medal winning book, put it with two other illustrated children's books that have not won the Caldecott Medal, and ask your pupil to choose which one she thinks has the best illustrations and won the medal. That is, suggest that your pupil pretend that she is one of the judges for the Caldecott Medal.

Your point is not to humiliate your pupil if she doesn't chose the book the ALA chose, but to use the "test" to talk about the three books, determine how the illustrations support the text, and so forth. It's also a good lesson in reading if you choose books with the simplest of texts.

If your child can't read one or all of the three books you choose, good to read each one aloud to your pupil, helping her to focus on the illustrations, and helping your pupil to make the connection between the illustrations—both how they are done and how they support the story.

The next step—"Garnish with the Arts throughout the Lessons"—will help you think of even more ways to build on your pupil's kinesthetic strengths.

IS THERE ANYTHING ELSE ABOUT USING STATISTICS?

The more you know about your pupil's interests, hobbies, special-interest activities, and the games she likes to play and/or watch, and the more you choose tutoring activities based on these interests, the more enthusiasm your pupil will show for doing the work necessary to gain fluency in reading and math.

Remember: You have guaranteed your pupil that you will teach him/her to read and do math.

Perhaps swimming is a special activity your pupil enjoys. If so, it would be good for the two of you to watch a swim team practice and if possible watch a competition. If possible, your pupil might be allowed to use a stopwatch and learn how to measure swimming time.

Out of this activity could come tables and graphs.

Or, it may be track and field activities. Again, securing information and creating tables and graphs are enormously helpful to a pupil to solidify her ability to read and write key words and terms.

I once used a pupil's fascination with an aquarium to help her develop excellent skill in creating artistic drawings of fish, snails, seaweed, and a hiding place. All she needed was drawing paper and colored pencils. She learned, as she drew, to label each item, checking in her dictionary (and with me, her tutor) to be sure the spelling was correct.

She wrote several stories. In one, a snail was the "voice." In another, it was a piece of seaweed complaining about being knocked over so often. In another, it was a Zebra fish complaining that it had no bright colors.

She illustrated each story, put them into a booklet, and gave the booklet to the first-grade classroom in her school after reading all the stories and showing the pictures to them.

YES! You can teach reading and math the kinesthetic way.

Step 7

Garnish with the Arts throughout the Lessons

WHOSE FAULT IS IT THAT YOUR PUPIL DIDN'T LEARN TO READ?

Essentially, it is the fault of the teaching your pupil received. If your pupil's family is illiterate and he was never read to during infancy and the toddler years, that contributed to the problem. If he came to school both hungry and physically tired, that contributed to the problem. If poor sight or poor hearing were difficulties, that contributed to the problem. If your pupil's family did not speak and read English in the home, that too contributed to the problem.

It is, however, in overwhelming numbers, the kinesthetic learner who fails to learn to read during those first three years of school. And that is not only because the teaching is done by those who learn visually or orally, but also because the teaching methods used by primary school teachers are geared almost exclusively to visual and oral learners.

The child with normal intelligence who needs and does not receive kinesthetic instruction day after day, month after month, and year after year is going to develop unhelpful behaviors. He's going to be his own worst literacy enemy. On top of this, he may be left-handed in a predominantly right-handed world. In fact, the majority of children who fail a third-grade reading test are left-handed.

You need to see through all the disruptive behaviors your pupil exhibits, recognizing that he really does want to be able to do what almost all of his classmates have learned to do—pass the reading tests he's given in grade 4. He didn't pass the reading tests he took in grade 1, grade 2, or grade 3. If he's going to have to repeat grade 3 if he fails the reading exams, the student absolutely wants to be able to pass the tests he's given. And if he is permitted to enter grade 4, he wants to pass the reading tests given in that grade.

Keep that in mind: your pupil wants to learn and is counting on you to show him how to do this. Therefore, you want to be sure you give him as many opportunities to learn by feeling as possible. And all the arts, because they include feeling and physical activity, will help you teach him and will help him learn how to learn.

You also want to help such a pupil learn how to work and play comfortably with others. Which sport would be better for your kinesthetic learner: archery or soccer? Not archery. First, one does it alone. Second, it's primarily visual, and all movement is prescribed. While soccer, on the other foot, involves moving something, somewhere as the result of thought and feeling. Also, soccer is played with a team, giving each player the opportunity to perform at a relatively similar level of ability.

HOW DO YOU INCLUDE DANCING IN THE LESSONS?

Dancing, like soccer, not only requires kinesthetic actions but also easily adapts to partners and groups. Also, dance steps can be diagrammed, first in the sand tray, then with the black crayon, in the air, on the chalkboard, and with steps chalked onto the floor. Start with ballroom dancing or with folk dancing. Just be sure that you help your pupil diagram how the steps should go.

Talk your pupil through the steps while demonstrating them and have your pupil copy the movements, but also be sure to have the pupil both draw and explain in written words what the feet should do.

You might not consider it dancing, but cheerleading requires movements that are wonderful activities for the kinesthetic learner. Again, cheerleading is an activity that puts nonreaders on equal ground with fellow pupils who are passing the reading tests. This won't be true, of course, if those who teach the cheerleaders hand out written materials describing what the athletes should do. If your pupil can first deal with a diagram, and with assistance make the movements shown in the diagrams, then he can be a productive member of the cheerleading team.

HOW DO YOU USE PHOTOGRAPHY IN THE LESSONS?

You will need access to a video camera.

What a wonderful way to tell a story! What a wonderful way to marry visual, oral, and kinesthetic learning styles! For example, you can help your pupil

- prepare a script and explain just what he wants his photography to depict. Then use the camera to follow the script.
- take a video and then develop the script that is depicted in the video.
- make a video of a dance routine. Along with the video, have your pupil write an accompanying script explaining what the video is showing.
- make a video of a cheerleading routine, then diagram the routine, describe the routine in written words, and prepare an oral script to go with the video.
- make a video of a team sport—five minutes, for example, of an

ice hockey or field hockey game. Then help your pupil write the script explaining the action he photographed. Teach him how to use what he has written to do an oral narration to accompany the video.

Even some of the math explorations and stories in step 6 can be photographed and shared with others interested in learning how to solve word problems.

HOW DO YOU USE DRAWING IN THE LESSONS?

If you aren't a skilled artist, perhaps you can locate a tutor who would teach your pupil some drawing skills. What about a college student studying art?

Most of the art teachers I've asked to help my pupils have started with charcoal and soft-lead pencils. From there, the pupils have quickly learned about shading and perspective.

They have loved not only doing the drawings to illustrate their "made-up" stories but also creating illustrated graphs depicting their math explorations.

Finger painting, as you might suspect, delights the kinesthetic learner. And most third and fourth graders are thrilled when they can use both watercolor and oil paints to create their drawings and paintings.

HOW DO YOU USE CLAY IN THE LESSONS?

- When you read a story to your pupil, give him some soft clay and suggest that while he's listening, he make a shape that illustrates in some way what he thinks about the story. If you

read *Make Way for Ducklings*, for example, you may get a clay duckling or pond.
- If it is at all possible, see to it that your pupil has access to a potter's wheel and someone to provide the instruction.
- Since your kinesthetic pupil is going to be good at working with clay, it would be useful to have him join a class where he can demonstrate success along with his fellow pupils. Remember, his failure to learn to read makes him think there is something wrong with him; his success in learning to shape clay will help him realize that there is nothing wrong with him.

HOW DO YOU USE POETRY IN THE LESSONS?

You particularly want to help your pupil memorize poems that tell a story and depict a scene. As mentioned earlier, "Hiawatha" was an inspiration for one third grader.

Today, there are a host of good poets writing for children. But poets writing for adults also create wonderful word images that help the kinesthetic learner.

Howard Nemerov's poem "Epigrams" has a glorious pair of verses retelling the story of "The Emperor's New Clothes":

Epigrams

They gathered shouting crowds along the road
To praise his Majesty's satin and cloth-of-gold
But "Naked! Naked!" the children cried.

Now when the gaudy clothes ride down the street
No child is found sufficiently indiscreet
To whisper "No majesty's inside."

This is just the type of twist children love. After sharing the original story and then Howard Nemerov's version, the next step might be to have your pupil compose his own poem about this famous naked majesty.

Then, too, children love to learn the lyrics of popular songs as well as folk music. Christmas carols, ballads, rounds, and hymns are marvelous sources, both for the read-aloud time, and for helping your pupil create his own verses.

> 💡 **Remember:** Tracing is necessary when learning song lyrics.

You might want to go with your pupil to a local school or public library, browse through the poetry section, and help your pupil choose one or two books of verse. Perhaps this is something parents or guardians will want to do.

For many a pupil, I've been asked to read aloud from countless books of poetry, hymnals, and folk song collections.

HOW DO YOU USE SINGING AND SHEET MUSIC IN THE LESSONS?

If you do not know how to read and write musical scores, perhaps you can hire someone who can tutor your pupil. What about a college student majoring in music composition?

What you want is someone who can listen to a few notes sung by your pupil, then score those sounds and help your pupil learn how to score his own musical sounds. It's often good for your pupil to listen to a piece of music, then write the score based on what he heard—and vice versa, if you pupil is faced with a score, he should work out how should it be played.

This is, as you well recognize, excellent for developing oral and aural skills. And what you are doing is offering your pupil the kinesthetic step—the writing of the sounds, not just the hearing of them.

If all you know is the scale and all you have is a recorder or an old upright piano, have your pupil learn how to write what he hears and be able, by looking at a score, to know what its sounds should be.

HOW DO YOU USE DRUMMING IN THE LESSONS?

Drumming is the perfect skill for a kinesthetic learner. If you don't know how to beat a snare drum or read the music guiding you to shake the bells or strike the cymbal, find a tutor who does know drumming to help your pupil. Is there a college student who plays in the marching band you could ask to help you tutor your pupil? You don't need a full orchestra; you can play a tape of a piece of stirring martial music and teach your pupil to do the drumming along with the members of the orchestra.

Clapping rhythms is as old as time, and it's an excellent activity for a kinesthetic learner. Teach your pupil how to read the music score that produces the rhythm to clap. Teach your pupil how to tap his feet and clap his hands to accompany marching music. Teach him to march to different music scores. And teach him to read those scores so that he can tell the difference in marching patterns because of the musical patterns.

HOW DO YOU USE A PUPPET SHOW IN THE LESSONS?

As you can imagine, using hand puppets to tell an original story—first dictated by, then read and written by, your pupil—will help him develop as a successful reader.

Turn a sock into a gorilla, and perform the puppet show "I saw a gorilla at the zoo." As your pupil progresses and his stories become more complicated, so may the puppet shows. And how wonderful to have an audience made up of preschoolers!

Is there someone who can help your pupil build a puppet show stage? Perhaps a college student interested in theater? Is there an older child who would be willing to be one of the other puppets?

Your pupil needs to be the one to dictate (and then write) the story. It is your pupil who should write the choreography directions for the staging, dialog, and music.

HOW DO YOU USE ACTING IN THE LESSONS?

Now this will take enormous tact on your part, but it will be well worth whatever it takes to accomplish it—your pupil needs to have a part in a play put on at school. It needs to be a speaking part, even if it's just one word or one phrase. And you need to help your pupil understand not only the full story but also the importance of all the stage directions.

All that goes in to understanding the play and its performance are perfect stimulants for the kinesthetic learner. Your pupil has to be somewhere and do something. Ideally, if there is a chorus, your pupil can be in it.

The very reason for using plays for schooling is to develop reading and speaking skills, yet, most often, only those pupils who pass the reading tests are given opportunities to perform for the public. The third-grade pupil who needs to be in a play is the one who is struggling to learn to read, not the one who already is proficient.

If your pupil does get into the play and the part he is to play is small enough that he can grasp it completely, the very circumstance of being successful in such a drama will do wonders for the pupil. It will, of course, do more to raise his reading test scores than it ever

Garnish with the Arts throughout the Lessons 109

will do for the reading scores of the pupils his age who have been reading since the middle of grade 1.

Even if your pupil doesn't get a speaking part, there are many ways the still-learning-to-read pupil can be part of a performance. And it is the performance as a whole that often helps the pupil understand yet another piece of the reading puzzle.

HOW IS BEING ON THE STAGE CREW USED IN THE LESSONS?

Often work on the stage crew is reserved for those pupils who don't need the activity to pass the reading test. And the very pupils whose learning style would be helped by serving on the stage crew are not given the opportunity. Pair the nonreader with a reader, if necessary, but see to it that the pupils having difficulty learning to read are the ones who have the opportunity to improve their construction abilities.

Don't just let them pound nails or saw boards. Use those activities for stories, and for tracing, and for learning the words that accompany stage directions.

If act 1 needs a bed and act 2 does not, have the student place the bed onstage and take it off, as this responsibility will make that pupil feel part of the production. The stage directions are very simple, easily read and understood by a kinesthetic pupil, and counting on this pupil to be sure that the bed is where it belongs on stage in act 1, and off the stage for act 2, is enormously important for any school that wants to make a reader of that pupil.

HOW DO YOU USE ARCHITECTURE AND DESIGN IN THE LESSONS?

- Teach your pupil how to draw the dimensions (cubic) of the room in which your teaching is taking place; it might be good

to use graph paper. Place the furniture on the floor plan for the room. Locate windows and doors and any outstanding features. Have the pupil do the measurements.
- Do drawings of other spaces. Teach an appreciation for use of space. Teach your pupil how to fill a space attractively and usefully.
- Choose a building in town that is architecturally important, and have your pupil do a drawing of the outside and of some of the interior rooms.
- Study a garden space, then help your pupil reproduce it on paper. Then ask your pupil to design his own garden space.
- Have your student design part of an elementary school playground.
- Have your student design a play area connected with a home.
- Have your student design a soccer field; a basketball court with benches for visitors; a softball field; an outdoor volleyball area. That is, have your pupil make these designs and add them to the three-hole notebook.
- With your pupil, study a garden space and create an exact design of that space. As you fill the space, teach the pupil the names for the flowers, bushes, trees, furniture, and so forth by tracing. Perhaps you could put a small bridge in this garden space; learning how to design a bridge may require asking for assistance from a college student taking engineering courses.

Supporting your pupil's natural artistic talent is most important. Singing, dancing, acting, drawing, and designing all make important use of the kinesthetic learning method. They all bring beauty and grace to the effort. How wonderful for your pupil to be able to balance the struggle to decipher words with the joy of expression.

Step 8

Stop Reading Aloud

At some point in your lessons, you want to stop reading aloud to your student. You want to do this while you are still helping her learn to read by tracing some words and while you are still helping her write her own stories.

You do want to stop reading a story to your pupil that your pupil wants very much to read, but you don't want to stop reading aloud too soon.

Let's posit that you are reading a mystery story and that your pupil is fully engaged in the story, eager to talk over what has already taken place, and while you are reading aloud, listens attentively. This is the ideal time to stop reading aloud—when your pupil is motivated to read on her own to find out what happens.

IS IT TIME FOR YOU TO STOP READING TO YOUR PUPIL?

Is it time for you to say, "Why don't you read it to yourself now?" How will you know when that is the right question to ask?

1. One measure that signifies your pupil might be ready to read on her own is that your pupil is no longer dictating her story but is writing it herself, asking you to help supply new words.

2. Another measure of progress is your pupil's ability to use her card file on her own initiative and her ability to use the dictionary to find a word that she needs.
3. Finally, you need to feel that your pupil trusts that your teaching is working; that she is, at last, succeeding at learning to read.

However, you do not want to stop reading to your pupil while she is still tentative about reading to herself. Yet if she decides to try reading to herself at this point, you need to "be there" for her, providing the pronunciation of a word, discussing its meaning, and able to recall what that particular story is about.

If it is a mystery, you need to have read the story carefully enough to know what is happening in the section your pupil is trying to read to herself. You want to be able to discuss elements of the story with your pupil both while she is reading (if she starts such a discussion) and after she has completed the reading for a single lesson period.

Of course, your pupil needs to have access to whatever it is she's reading whether she's having the tutoring lesson or not. Even if it's a nonfiction article in a reference book, she should, if it is possible, have it available for her to look at and read 24/7.

And you need to be able to review the material so that you can discuss it intelligently with your student and help her think through how to use the material for writing her own stories, illustrating or creating a poem, making something with clay, or turning part of the text into a script for a play or skit.

SHOULD YOUR PUPIL READ THE STORY TO YOU?

If you are sure that what you are reading aloud during the final session of a lesson is something your pupil is really loving and enjoying, and you think she is progressing well enough that she needs to face the challenge of reading to herself, let your pupil try it. Sit close by so you can tell if you have required too soon that your pupil do her own reading, that is, if she loses interest in the material fairly quickly.

Offer to read a few paragraphs aloud yourself, then ask her to read a few paragraphs aloud to you. And when that seems to be working, suggest that she read her paragraphs to herself, then you read aloud the next few paragraphs, then she reads a few more paragraphs silently, and after a period of time sharing in this manner, discuss what has happened in the story deeply enough so you know whether she has accurately read the material during the time she was reading to herself.

Generally, the optimum time to wean your pupil from listening to you read a story is when you are in the middle of the story, or part way through a document. My "D" encyclopedia pupil took over his own reading when we got to "dam." First he asked me to read aloud, but then he asked if he could just read it himself.

He read about dams. He memorized names and volumes in cubic yards of dams. He drew dams. He constructed dams. He talked about dams with family members and elders in the community. (Too bad your pupil doesn't live in Townshend, Vermont, where, near a real dam, is the Dam Diner serving a Dam Good Hamburger.)

My pupil dictated story after story under the same title: "The Dam Story." And his family reported that he had been scouring the shelves of their local public library to learn more about dams.

I wanted another one of my pupils to get as interested in fiction as he was in nonfiction, so I suggested he look up the name "Dickens, Charles." When I read to him that this author was "most popular" and "greatest," he asked me to read something written by him during our reading period. I did, and half way through Dickens's *A Christmas Carol*, I stopped reading aloud and suggested he finish the story himself.

But Dickens's books were not to his liking, so he continued finding nonfiction material that he did want to read to himself, with help from me for understanding words and particularly for discussing the information he was collecting.

SHOULD YOUR PUPIL READ ALOUD TO YOUNGER CHILDREN?

It is very helpful at this transition time to make available to your pupil a great number of easy-to-read books that she might choose to read aloud to an infant or toddler. If the family does not have a younger child available, suggest visits to local nursery schools and kindergartens.

This, too, is an enormous boost for your pupil. As soon as she can read from a published book, not just her own compositions, she should be given the opportunity to read aloud to an appreciative audience. In so doing, she gains skill in reading and strengthens her belief that she can read; she now can do what her fellow classmates learned to do.

WHAT ABOUT READING A PLAY TOGETHER?

Another step in helping your pupil gain both skill and confidence in reading aloud is to read a play together. You may need to read all but one of the parts and have your pupil read just one, but that one part should, of course, be the main character.

Some pupils will want to read the stage directions and actually be interested in depicting how the play can be staged.

Here is a grand opportunity for your pupil to diagram the stage area for the play you are reading. It also would be excellent for your pupil to list the props needed and to work out the scheme for the set design for each scene.

Stop Reading Aloud

HOW IS THE TUTORING SESSION ADAPTING TO YOUR PUPIL'S PROGRESS?

1. You are still going to start each lesson by asking your pupils what words she wants to learn by tracing. She is going to add those words to her card file.
2. You are going to help her write a new story on scrap paper. You are still going to be the one to make sure that the typed version of the story has no grammatical errors, no spelling errors, suitable punctuation, and, if appropriate, subheadings. You will ask your pupil to note the differences between the version written by her on the scrap paper and the corrected, typed version.
3. You are going to type the story, listing below it, in alphabetical order, all new words. You are going to help your pupil learn those new words by tracing and then by placing them in her card file.
4. Your pupil is going to illustrate a freshly typed version of the story without the lists of words to learn.
5. You are going to listen to your pupil read her story and explain her illustrations. You may have a separate audience available to hear her new story and see her illustrations.
6. You may encourage your pupil to practice old dance steps or learn a new dance step. You may sing a new or old song. You may help your pupil to begin designing a puppet show.
7. Then you will teach your pupil to do some interesting math exploration, possibly working on a video exploring a math concept. You'll help your pupil work on a word problem with a math base. Your pupil will use her counting items to depict math concepts. She will take measurements and find geometric spaces in the area you are using for the tutoring sessions, both inside and outside.
8. You will have had at least two recess periods during each lesson time, and during the final time, both of you will read to

yourselves. Maybe you will take turns reading aloud with your pupil, but maybe, too, she's ready to read to herself, gaining an understanding of the reading by discussing it with you.

WHAT AREN'T YOU GOING TO DO?

1. *You are never going to say,*

"We learned that yesterday."
"You should know that; we already traced it."
"Why are you asking me the same question today?"
"You haven't been paying attention and that's why you . . ."
"I can't teach you; you're not trying."
"You probably can't learn this dance step; it's very difficult."
"You are going to keep tracing this until you get it right."
"It's not my fault you didn't learn it."
"You should be ashamed that you haven't learned this yet."
"I am only going to give you baby books to read."
"Why didn't you memorize that?"

2. *You are never going to teach homonyms in the same lesson.* "Bore" and "boar" sound the same, but they don't have the same meaning or spelling. For the kinesthetic learner, they are best taught in separate lessons and best presented when the context is helpful. For the visual learner, it would be fun to study this sentence:

<blockquote>Your boar story is such a bore.</blockquote>

I have heard it too many times.

That's not a helpful way for either the oral or kinesthetic learners to be taught. When either of them hears the word "boar," they want to see the animal.

3. *You are never going to use "boar" to give a phonics lesson based on the boat paddle, the "oar."* Or (pun intended) a phonics

lesson based on the "ore" that is a natural combination of minerals. And you won't want to show that "soar" belongs in one phonics list, and "sore" in another.

You will be tempted to do this, but don't!

Your pupil needs to come to this type of wordplay only after she's a fluent reader. And only if she thinks it is a good way for her to learn the spelling and meaning of words.

But, suppose the word "boar" comes in the reading or your pupil wants to learn it in the tracing session. Then it is a good time to introduce some of those words that have "oar" in the base. Also, it is a good time to take such a word as "soar" and teach the variations of the verb "to soar." Your pupil might trace four of them: "soar," "soared," "soars," and "soaring." Be sure that your pupil places each of these verbs in a sentence; use the scrap paper.

WHAT ABOUT GIVING YOUR PUPIL THE STANDARD READING TESTS?

Yes and no.

It may be mandated, and so you have no choice. If during the time you are doing the tutoring the school your pupil attends has all its pupils take achievement tests, your pupil is included.

You can ready her for this experience. Explain whether guessing is a good idea or not. If scores on wrong answers are subtracted from scores on correct answers, then guessing is counterproductive. But if the score comes only from the answers that are correct, guessing is an excellent idea.

Some standard reading tests are designed to be diagnostic. They are designed to tell you what about learning to read is positive for your pupil, and what is not. Such a diagnostic test can be a great help to the teacher who recognizes that the exam is really testing his teaching ability and not his pupil's learning ability.

Have you, in fact, helped your pupil know what to do when faced with a word she does not recognize?

Have you, in fact, helped your student know how to review a sentence or more to determine the context for unknown words?

And so on. By reviewing what your pupil does on a reading test, you will learn what you should do to improve your teaching.

By giving a series of tests you are able to note progress. I was part of a team of three tutors working for six weeks with the same six elementary school pupils who had failed tests in both math and reading. We tested the students each week, and we met daily to talk about what we were doing and how well we thought we were succeeding.

The test questions were of the same value but not identical, so it was possible to record failure or progress. Five of the students were moving up the scale with each test, and one was not improving—at least as shown by the tests.

The high point of this one student's life, so far, was being the number one pitcher on a winning little league baseball team. He was short in stature and very concerned about it. Two of his teachers began using baseball terms and activities for his tutoring, and I found a marvelous story about a boy named "Wacky" who wrote in the first person about how good it was to be "the small boy."

At the same time, this boy found a baby squirrel whose mother had been run over by a car and decided he would try to keep it alive by feeding it baby formula. In two weeks' time, with his test results soaring, the student had interviewed squirrel experts at two zoos and had begun reading a doctor's thesis on what to do to help the baby squirrel.

The tracing, the writing of the stories, the statistic record, and the reading-aloud time were all coordinated.

At the end of five weeks, the infant squirrel took off up a tall Coulter Pine tree, came down only once to accept some seed from his foster parent, and the following day went on his own. I knew my pupil was doing the same to me. He was not going to turn back, and my "thanks" was in the doing.

Step 9

Support Your Pupil's Success

WHEN SHOULD YOUR PUPIL GO BACK INTO THE REGULAR CLASSROOM?

Of course, each pupil is different from every other. While all the nonreading third and fourth graders may need similar—if not identical—teaching techniques to unlock for them the ability to read, success rates vary. Also, both the family and schooling circumstances are dissimilar, if not unique, for each emerging reader.

It may be the ideal situation to remove a pupil from school altogether and only involve him in tutoring lessons that teach him to learn to read via the kinesthetic method. Even after a pupil shows signs of beginning to read fairly normally, puzzling out the sounding of words and demonstrating an ability to write stories made up of a strong vocabulary and using acceptable grammar and spelling, it may be best for that pupil to continue with tutoring. You wouldn't want to put a pupil back into a classroom situation where once again, because he is being taught inappropriately, he is not able to keep up with the class.

Or it might be better for your pupil to participate in all third- or fourth-grade activities and continue the kinesthetic tutoring after school, on weekends, and during holidays in order to support and reinforce emerging success in reading and writing.

And very often it is necessary for your pupil to be tested by an expert who can not only assess achievement skills in basic school subjects but also estimate the degree of ability your pupil can bring to his studies. For example, one boy who was failing miserably in all his classes was classified by his teachers, the school administrators, and the school district's testing officials as below average in both achievement and ability. When he was given a battery of tests by an independent specialist, he was found to be in the lowest tenth percentile for comprehension, but in the highest tenth percentile for ability.

Yet when his kinesthetic tutoring began to be successful, his teachers who had previously given him encouraging remarks on his report card began skipping the remarks, simply giving him failing grades. Yes, they acknowledged to his parents, he had not been able to read at all at the beginning of grade 4 and now, three months into tutoring, he was reading at the second-grade level, but since he was in class with all fourth graders, they argued, it was important for him and his family to know that he was failing fourth grade.

After the school officials reviewed with his parents and the tutor the results of the independent testing and accepted the fact that they had not recognized his innate intellectual abilities, the boy stayed in school, his teachers stopped giving him failing grades, his tutoring continued, and by the end of grade 4, he was passing all comprehensive tests at the top level. But his academic teachers and school officials nearly undid what was being so carefully done.

This is an extremely fragile time for struggling learners. It is humiliating, frustrating, debilitating, enervating, eviscerating, deadening, even crippling for these children to fail, year after year, at a skill apparently so easy to learn that other children—who don't appear to be smarter at all sorts of other activities—succeed as readers and writers when they fail to do so.

On top of that, here they are in tutoring sessions, just beginning to understand how to read and write, yet they realize and worry about the fact that they are some 30,000 to 40,000 words behind their peers. They need all the encouragement that can be provided;

scorn from school officials or family members is, to say the least, counterproductive.

WHO SHOULD DECIDE THE MIX BETWEEN SCHOOL AND TUTORING?

The mix has to be negotiated, but it is the parents who know their child better than any tutor, schoolteacher, or education official.

It is also true, that once a nonreader discovers he can read, he is particularly conscious of what teaching is the most helpful. A family who tried to force a son to learn to read by refusing to let him play on a club baseball team until he was "up to grade level," removed from him the very activity that made him willing to try to learn to read. He was the best pitcher in the club. The boy's tutor started his reading lessons by reading the sports pages in the newspaper covering the teams he knew and helped his family see how important it was for him to continue playing baseball.

Another lad, who loved music and had learned to pluck a zither, started his road to reading by learning to read music scores and visualize what he heard and created with his fingers. For months, he went to school for a half-day and worked with both a kinetic tutor and a music teacher the other half. The transition to book reading was slow but came in a rush when it did come.

Thus, parents and tutors need to provide each pupil with the right mix of "normal" schooling and "special" tutoring.

Parents: Don't be intimidated by the school authorities. No one on earth knows your child better than you do. Even if a parent can

---

Here's the success rule: Make sure what you do is what's best for your pupil.

neither read nor write in any language, that parent knows what his child needs in order to learn how to read and write. Such illiterate parents cannot do the teaching, but they can insist that the school authorities provide the best teachers using the method most appropriate for their child.

HOW SHOULD YOU TEACH NOTE TAKING?

Pupils who learn visually can be shown how to use a florescent highlighter to help recall the most important words and phrases.

Pupils who learn orally can be shown how to pick out and read aloud words and phrases that carry the main message.

If your pupil learns kinesthetically, teach him how to take notes by writing the words and phrases that others might highlight or voice.

Let me give an example. I have taken some material from a workbook used by third, fourth, and fifth graders in the state of Vermont.

Example

French and Indian War

Lake Champlain was an important area for forts to be built and battles to be fought because it was both a major invasion route and supply route. Navigating boats on waterways was the fastest, easiest way to move armies and heavy things like cannons, food, and other supplies from place to place.

Using the St. Lawrence River, the Richelieu River, and Lake Champlain was like taking the back way into Vermont, New York, and Massachusetts. Starting from the Hudson River and taking short portages (places where you had to carry your boat overland) drops one right into Lake Champlain, which is the route into Canada. So naturally, the Native Americans, British, French, and Americans all fought for control of this route.

> During several periods of the 1600s and 1700s, the British were at war with France. Of course, that meant both the British colonies in America and New France (Canada) were involved in the wars.
> One war between the British and French started in 1755 and lasted seven years. It is known as the French and Indian War or the Seven Years' War. Lake Champlain was a scene of great activity. Armies from both sides traveled its length.

A good many teachers want nothing more from third and fourth graders than recall of names, dates, and events from the reading of such a typical selection. A tutor would have a pupil write the name of the selection, the names of the lake and the three rivers, and the fact that the war was between Britain and France and between the American and Canadian colonies. The dates—1600s, 1700s, and 1755—would also be written.

But let's suppose the questions would be more probing, for example,

- Why did the British and the French in the 1600s and 1700s build forts on the shores of Lake Champlain?
- What is the water route from Canada to New York using the St. Lawrence River?
- What is a portage?
- Why did the colonialists in America and Canada fight each other?

As you ask each question, have your pupil write the answer—not necessarily using complete sentences but clearly noting the key information. To answer the second question about the water route, it would help the kinesthetic learner to look on a map and to run a finger up and down from Canada to New York. You should also have your pupil find the names of the bodies of water, as well as Vermont, New York, and Massachusetts, on the map.

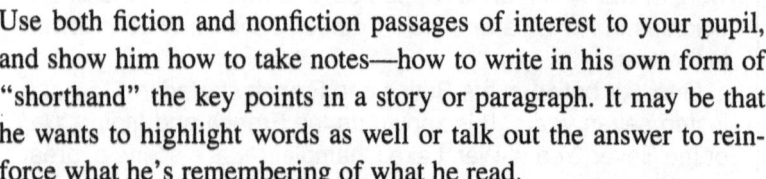

Use both fiction and nonfiction passages of interest to your pupil, and show him how to take notes—how to write in his own form of "shorthand" the key points in a story or paragraph. It may be that he wants to highlight words as well or talk out the answer to reinforce what he's remembering of what he read.

You might read a selection together, and ask your pupil to give the quiz about facts as well as general information. Ask him to write the questions, and you answer them in written form.

For the early lessons, always have the selection available to be read and reread by your pupil. But gradually try to teach him to read a selection, taking notes as he does so, then use only the notes to answer your questions about the selection.

HOW SHOULD YOU TEACH VOCABULARY?

The following information may include words that most third and fourth graders do not know; at the same time, the information is interesting to them, and something they should learn.

Examples

Right of Way—Sailing Vessels

- Vessel on *port tack* must give way to vessel on *starboard tack*.
- When two vessels are on the same tack, the windward vessel has right of way.
- When one vessel overtakes another, the vessel overtaken has right of way.
- Sailing vessel under power must give way to vessel under sail alone.

Only a few pupils will know most of the words in this rule of law for sailors. Again, because your pupil is a kinesthetic learner, it would be good to use toy ships or erasers or checker pieces and play out each of the laws.

Port, starboard, and windward—after being located in a dictionary—are good words to trace and add to the card file. Also, it's good for your pupil to pick out port and starboard sides of items in the classroom, or in a picture, or when graphing the meeting of two sailing boats.

While the pupil is demonstrating the rules, have him state the rules; just as you had your pupil say a word when tracing the word in the sand or on the black crayon writing.

The following rule involving a steam vessel and a sailing vessel would be an excellent one to have your pupil demonstrate, then restate in his own words. Or, have your pupil commit the rule to memory as it appears here. Remember, couple the gathering of information from a written text with as much tactile evidence as you can use to help in both recall and comprehension.

Right of Way—Steam Vessels

When a steam vessel and a sailing vessel are proceeding in such directions as to involve risk of collision, the steam vessel shall keep out of the way of the sailing vessel, *but* a sailing vessel has no right to hamper, in a narrow channel, the safe passage of a steam vessel that can navigate only inside that channel.

Again, help the pupil "see" what is happening. Perhaps you could use graph paper to depict how these rules apply. Or use toy boats to create the opportunity to demonstrate the "right of way." And remember to assist the pupil in making a note about this rule to help commit it to memory.

Vocabulary words could include the following:

right of way
proceeding (proceed, proceeded)
risk (risks, risking, risked)
collision (collisions)
hamper (hampers, hampering, hampered)
navigate (navigates, navigating, navigated)

This is a marvelous group of words, the meanings of which can come straight out of the pupil's demonstration of how this "right of way" rule would work. Again, trace each word if necessary and add to the card file. But don't neglect to give your pupil the opportunity to "feel" and "see" what each word means, not just in this context, but also in multiple uses.

～

You will remember that during the early lessons, you were told that it is not helpful for a kinesthetic learner to try to learn to spell and know the meanings of words that sound alike but have very different meanings; for example, "him" and "hymn." That's an easy lesson for a visual learner but a difficult one for both the oral and kinesthetic learner.

But you can combine vocabulary and spelling lessons for your kinesthetic learner by starting with a base word. Take the word "ball," for example. Once it is traced and made part of the known vocabulary, then its variations can be easily learned: football, baseball, soccer ball, ping pong ball, volley ball, tennis ball, softball, and so on. Using drawings or actual balls, provide your pupil with the feel of the object as well as the word.

Start with root words, such as "ship." With the dictionary for assistance, find "ships," "shipped," and "shipping." Again, play out in words and objects a ship, many ships, shipping activities, and so forth.

Over and over and over, tie a "thing" with a "thought" with a "word."

HOW SHOULD YOU TEACH COMPREHENSION?

In a word—dialogue.

Examples

Have your pupil read a paragraph silently, one you already know; then ask him questions about the material in the paragraph. First, limit yourself to yes-and-no questions. For example, go back to the "Right of Way—Steam Vessels" passage (p. 124):

In open water does the steam vessel have the right of way?
In a narrow channel does the steam vessel have the right of way?

Have your pupil take a comprehension test. Ask your pupil to show you the answer to the following question: Why does the steam vessel have the right of way in a narrow channel?

Play it out on graph paper, or with objects simulating the two vessels, perhaps even using a sink or tub full of water.

By now, you understand that it is the creating of the scene that is so important for the kinesthetic learner. And this, of course, is what leads you as tutor to help your pupil take a part in a play.

Start out by making your own plays using the stories your pupil has written during the first lessons. "The Gorilla at the Zoo" was, of course, the first play I did with that pupil. We did several plays in the zoo atmosphere based on his storytelling. And then we used a portion of *The Wind in the Willows* (by Kenneth Grahame) with each of us taking turns reading parts.

But we didn't just read the parts. We read what it was we were to say, but then we talked about the scene (and scenery), the conditions, our feelings, and what the dialogue meant; then we reviewed how the dialogue fit with the rest of the play; then we said our lines. And often, after reading some more of the play silently, we worked again on an earlier dialogue, determining just what we wanted the lines to convey.

We read the same passage to make the meaning happy, then sad.

And with most pupils there has been considerable joy producing a short play from a favorite poem.

~

Another stimulant to comprehension is to ask your pupil, once he has understood a moment in history—for example, President Lincoln's address at Gettysburg—to pretend that Lincoln gave the speech when television was available and that your pupil was the local news announcer assigned by the station manager to go to the cemetery in Gettysburg and report on Lincoln's speech.

Or, you be the announcer and let your pupil take the role of Lincoln. Or, you be the announcer and let your pupil takes the role of a wounded Union soldier who you interview about what happened.

Ask your pupil to picture how this play might look on the stage. Have him mentally construct the stage and the props. Do this with all plays; make your pupil the stage manager, maybe also the lighting manager. Your pupil's wonderful skill at creating a scene to which dialogue can be added will not only make the lesson a pleasure, but will also reinforce his ability to read new words, understanding them from their context.

~

Both you and your pupil will recognize the time for you to part. A handshake or "high-five" will do it for your pupil. But for you, the tutor, this is the beginning of another beginning. I am a big fan of Irma Rombauer's *Joy of Cooking*. Let me close by quoting from her introduction in my 1953 edition: "Your first efforts at cooking may result in confusion, but soon you will acquire a skilled routine that will give you confidence and pleasure."

Yes, your first efforts at teaching a kinesthetic learner may result in confusion, but following the directions in this recipe book for tutors, you really will acquire the knowledge and skill you need that will give you confidence and pleasure.

www.ingramcontent.com/pod-product-compliance
Lightning Source LLC
Chambersburg PA
CBHW021846220426
43663CB00005B/422